Chinese Ocular Diagnosis and Periocular Acupuncture

Compiled by
Hoy Ping Yee Chan, O.M.D.

with expanded material from
Y. M. Chen, Ph.D. (OM), L.Ac.

AyniWrite Press
10700 Academy Rd NE #2227 Albuquerque, NM 87111
www.AyniWritePress.com

Chinese Ocular Diagnosis and Periocular Acupuncture / Chan and Chen -- 1st Ed
ISBN 978-0-9907550-1-2

Window of Health
Golden Words
to Our Dear Readers

There is an old Chinese saying, "*The eye is the window of the soul*". From the expression and brightness of the eye, we can see through to a person's mind, like one can see inside a house through the windows. Hence, where the title of this book, *The Window of Health - Ocular Diagnosis and Periocular Acupuncture* came from. Through the knowledge contained in this book, we will be able to recognize the health condition of a person. Since the eye is the mirror of the soul and also reflects the health condition of the body, this old Chinese saying is as important and true today as it was when it was written.

Dedication

This book is dedicated to Professor Peng Jingshan's Ocular Acupuncture Research Department of Liaoning College of Traditional Chinese Medicine and to the Northwest Institute of Acupuncture and Oriental Medicine in the United States of America.

Acknowledgments

Honorable appreciation to Alex Holland, L.Ac., Robert Lanphear, Rebekah Everett, Cindy Nash, Lydia Sterling, Yuanming Lu, L.Ac., Diane Williams and Dina Chan for their contribution to the success of this book. Special thanks to the Northwest Institute of Acupuncture and Oriental Medicine for publishing this book as the first of all their publications.

Table of Contents

Golden Words to Our Dear Readers iii

Dedication and Acknowledgments iv

Forward ix

Preface to *Window of Health* 1st Ed xi

Introduction to *Window of Health* 1st Ed xiii

CHAPTER ONE

Historical Review 1

1. Classical Writings 1
2. About the Inventor 2

CHAPTER TWO

Relative Anatomy 5

1. The Superficial Look and Skin of Palpebrae 5
2. The Muscles 6
3. The Sensory Nerve 8
4. The Circulation 9
5. The Distribution of Nerves and Arteries in the Deeper Layer of Each Periocular Region 11

CHAPTER THREE

Theory 13

1. The Eye and Meridians 13
2. The Eye and Muscle Regions 21
3. The Eye and Organs (Zang-Fu) 22
4. The Five Phases and Five Wheels 28
5. The Eight Diagrams and Eight Octants 28

CHAPTER FOUR

Location 33

1. The Thirteen Ocuzones 33
2. Triple-Warmer Theory 34
3. The Location 36

CHAPTER FIVE

Disease Recognition 39

1. Pathological Variances in the Capillary Branches of the Bulbar Conjunctiva 39
2. Color Variances in the Capillary Branches 42
3. Results of a Double Blind Study in Observation of Ocular Diagnosis 42

CHAPTER SIX

Therapy 43

1. The Principle of Selection 43
2. The Indications and Therapeutic Prescriptions from Dr. Peng's Experience 45
3. Experiences of Other Acupuncturists 50
4. Personal Experience - Complicated Symptoms 50

CHAPTER SEVEN

Periocular Needling Technique 51

1. Insertion 51
2. The Various Puncturing Methods 51
3. Needle Manipulation 55
4. Needle Retention 55
5. Withdrawal of Needle 55
6. Contraindications 55
7. Tips on the Method 55
8. Ten Precautionary Measures 56

CHAPTER EIGHT
Clinical Reports 59

1. Professor Peng's Report of 13 Typical Cases 59
2. Periocular Acupuncture for Cholecyspasm 62
3. Clinical Research on Ocular Diagnosis and Periocular Acupuncture 63
4. Ocular Diagnosis and Periocular Acupuncture for Complicated Symptoms 64
5. Clinical Reports from Author Hoy Ping Yee Chan, OMD 68

CHAPTER NINE
Prevention: Periocular Self Care 71

1. Periocular Acupressure by Finger 71
2. A Smooth Round Tip Probe 71
3. A Ferrite Magnet 72
4. A Magnetic Blunt Tip Needle 72

References 73

About the Author 75

Addendum by Dr. Y.M. CHEN 77

1. Based Evidence of Chinese Medicine for Eyes 1
2. What Chinese Medicine Says About Our Eyes 2
3. Five Types of Eyes 2
4. Secondary Eye Dysfunctions 2
5. Key Words and Abbreviations 3
6. Diagnosis and Treatment for Five Types of Eye Dysfunction 3
7. Special Discussion: Periocular Acupuncture Dx and Tx for Post Traumatic Injury Syndrome (PTIS) and Stroke............. 15
8. Chinese Periocular Acupuncture with Chinese Periocular Tuina 18
9. Twelve Important Prevention Measures for Your Eye Care 22
10. Five Pathogenic Factors that Affect Our Eyes Daily 25

11. Five Impairments by Five Prolonging or Reparative Motions 26
12. How Ocuzones and Acupuncture Points Relate to Eye Dysfunction 26
13. More Evidence Based Findings 27

References 30

Ocuzone Charts 33

Special Thanks 34

Forward

Periocular Acupuncture is another very special modality of micro-acupuncture, created in 1970 by Professor Peng Jingshan, from Liaoning College of TCM. It has been promoted and developed in the USA and other countries in the world by many of Professor Peng's students. One of those students was Dr. Hoy Ping Yee Chan, OMD, NCCA Diplomat of Acupuncture and Herbology (Retired), from Washington State. In 1993 Dr. Chan studied in Professor Peng's Eye Needle Therapy clinic (眼針療法門診部). She dedicated herself and practiced this therapy for so many years at her greater Seattle office. Her first book *Window of Health*, published in 1996, has helped many acupuncturists understand basic principles, diagnosis, and treatment methods of Professor Peng's Eye Needle Therapy used for stroke rehabilitation, neurological impairment, internal disorders and pain relief. Also this technique is very effective for many eye diseases such as degenerative eye dysfunctions that affect all ages.

Many of my own patients ranging from 12 to 85 years old have received periocular acupuncture treatments and have shown positive outcomes from this method. Some of my patients have even experienced restored vision and maintained eye wellbeing for a long period of time without any reduction of their eyesight through the preventive use of Periocular Acupuncture and Periocular Tuina. These therapies have helped patients with conditions such as eye allergies, Bell's palsy, cataracts, dry eye syndrome, ocular migraine, photophobia, myopia, diabetic retinopathy, retinitis pigmentosa (night blindness), glaucoma, macular degeneration and stroke. In this digital age this treatment approach especially helped those with Digital Eye Dysfunction (DED) or Computer Vision Syndrome (CVS), providing a balanced treatment for both mental and ocular yin/yang imbalance from prolonged use of computers, playing online games, cell phone texting and watching TV. CPA is also recognized clinically as another treatment approach for both neuromuscular and internal medicine issues because ocular manifestation occurs depending on the metastasis of each affected organ.

Many evidenced-based studies indicate that diabetes, hypertension, allergies, brain tumor, stroke, cystic fibrosis, head trauma, leukemia, or thyroid disease can cause serious eye problems. As a matter of fact, ocular melanoma or cancer is one of the major concerns in our society now.

A special thanks to Dr. Chan's years of research and promotion of ocular diagnosis and periocular acupuncture in the USA. Her contribution is greatly appreciated by our community and each practitioner who currently uses this therapy.

In the addendum of this book, I will share my years of personal experience in the field of Chinese Periocular Acupuncture and Periocular Tuina as well as preventive care. I sincerely hope that my findings and treatment protocols will help others who are interested in these particular methods to improve diagnosis and produce more effective results. Thus, Chinese Periocular Acupuncture and Periocular Tuina will continue to be discussed, practiced, promoted, restored and developed from generation to generation throughout the world.

Y.M. Chen, Ph.D. (OM), L.Ac.

President of Chinese Health Center

Anthem, AZ, U.S.A.

Preface to *Window of Health, 1st Ed.*

Acupuncture is an important component of traditional Chinese medicine. This preventative and healing therapy has been accepted by the Chinese and other Asians for thousands of years. Micro-acupuncture, as a branch of acupuncture science, has expanded rapidly throughout the world in the recent half century. Ocular Diagnosis and Periocular Acupuncture is the youngest therapeutic tool of the micro-acupuncture system. It was invented by Professor Peng Jingshan in 1970. Clinical research using this unique method on 10,000 patients, recognized disease by observing the eye for diagnosis and showed a 90% accuracy rate.

I first explored this therapy in 1987 at the "First World Conference on Acupuncture-Moxibustion", which was held in Beijing, China. Since then, I have collected available information to learn more about this technique, but until Professor Jingshan's book *Ocular Acupuncture Therapy* was published in November of 1990, there was little information to be found.

I did go ahead and add this therapy to my practice, but felt it would be beneficial to learn firsthand how ocular diagnosis and periocular acupuncture was actually practiced on patients. In 1993, I went to Liaoning College of Traditional Chinese Medicine to study in Professor Peng's Ocular Therapy Research Department. The doctors and patients of the department reported remarkable and beneficial results from using this technique for pain relief and stroke rehabilitation. I was very impressed with the results and expressed my goal to them: after I returned to the United States, I would like to introduce this successful therapy to my colleagues and patients. I thank the National Acupuncture and Oriental Medicine Alliance for giving me the chance to introduce Ocular Diagnosis and Periocular Acupuncture at the conference held in Seattle, Washington in May of 1996.

This book is a compilation of Professor Peng's work, *Ocular Needle Therapy*, which is printed in Chinese, and the lecture on "Ocular Acupuncture *(Part 1 and 2)*" in the 1993 *International Journal of Clinical Acupuncture*, Volume 4, Nos.1 and 2.

Special thanks to the Foreign Languages Press of Bejing, China for giving me permission to use eighteen illustrations from the book, *Chinese Acupuncture and Moxibustion*. These pictures are to help the reader to better understand the close relationship between the eye, the meridians and the body.

I will continue to learn and practice this new therapy and hope for the chance to do more research. I look forward to the day when the first ocular diagnosis and periocular acupuncture conference is held in the United States. It will provide a forum for the discussion and sharing of the benefits of this unique technique, as other branches of micro-acupuncture have done; a day when more acupuncturists see the benefits of ocular diagnosis and periocular acupuncture for their patients and feel comfortable using this technique in their practice. Please remember, it is always better to have one more tool at work and holding one more key while trying to open a door. Thank you for reading this book. Any comments are welcome.

Hoy Ping Yee Chan, L.Ac., O.M.D.

Seattle, Washington

November 1996

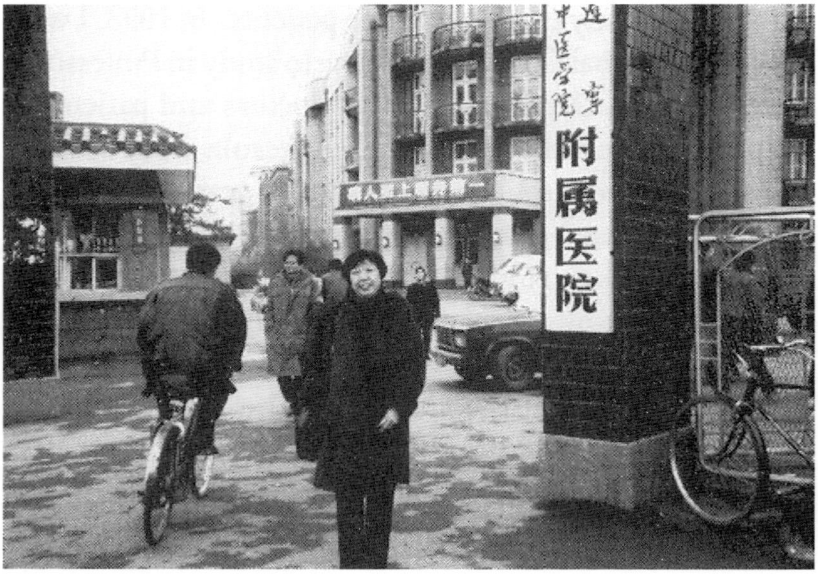

Figure 1 Hoy Ping Yee Chan at the Entrance of the Outpatient Department of the Hospital of Liaoning College of TCM in 1993

Introduction to *Window of Health, 1st Ed.*

This book is intended as a guide to the clinical application of a new Chinese microsystem, the orbit of the eye, and its usage through ocular diagnosis and periocular acupuncture. Traditional Chinese medicine has a long and evolved history out of which has developed the highly refined skill of empirical observation. The blending of these two, history and observation, has resulted in the development of a number of microsystems which use the principles upon which Oriental medicine was founded. Chinese clinical experience, spanning centuries, coupled with a deep understanding of meridian energetics, has fostered a continual search for new ways to stimulate healing. The new microsystem incorporated in Ocular Diagnosis and Periocular Acupuncture is the most recent of these developments.

Ocular Acupuncture Therapy utilizes the microsystem which encircles the eye and was developed by Dr. Peng Jingshan over the past 25 years. This system of diagnosis and treatment is fast gaining international recognition as a simple and effective means employing acupuncture to assist the body in the healing process. This book was designed for those individuals who are already practicing acupuncture and want to expand their therapeutic options.

Ocular Diagnosis and Periocular Acupuncture stems from a holistic understanding of the body and as such is similar to other microsystems used in traditional Chinese medicine. Each microsystem is unique in its ability to stimulate healing and each has specific applications in conjunction with other modalities which reinforce the healing effects. Ocular Diagnosis and Periocular Acupuncture, although an effective treatment in its own right, is a new enough modality to warrant thoughtful research to help determine its true strengths in relation to other more traditional treatment strategies and techniques. As a system of healing in China, it has shown promise in a number of diseases which were difficult to treat using other means.

The Northwest Institute wishes to thank Dr. Hoy Ping Yee Chan for her dedicated work in this field and for helping to bring this valuable new form of Oriental medical treatment to the acupuncture profession in the United States.

Alex Holland, M.Ac., L.Ac.
Northwest Institute of Acupuncture and Oriental Medicine

CHAPTER ONE

Historical Review

Ocular diagnosis and periocular acupuncture is one form of micro-system acupuncture. It is based on traditional Chinese medical theory and as stated in *Plain Questions*, "All channels converge at the eye". It is possible to recognize health conditions by observing the eye and to treat diseases by needling the points around the eye.

Classical Writings

In traditional Chinese medicine, the relationship between the eye and the body (Zang-Fu) was already written about in the *Yellow Emperor's Canon of Internal Medicine*.

"The five Zang and six Fu essences flow into the eye and nourishes it."- *Big Questions, Miraculous Pivot.*

"The 12 channels and 365 collaterals, Blood and Qi flow upward into the head and its orifices. Its Yang Qi essence flows into the eye and nourishes it."- *The Pathology of Evils in Zang-Fu, Miraculous Pivot.*

Hua Tuo said, "The eye's form is like a sphere. Its' pupil is centered in front like the sun and moon shining from the southeast to northwest. Included are six large channels: Heart, Lung, Spleen, Liver, Kidney and Mingmen. Each large channel has its own special function: eight channels in between, consisting of the Gallbladder, Stomach, Large and Small Intestine, Triple-Jiao (Upper Warmer, Middle Warmer and Lower Warmer) and Urinary Bladder. There are many fine collaterals which flow downward, passing through the brain and connecting with the Zang-Fu below, aiding the coming and going of Qi and Blood to vitalize the eye. If disease occurs, specific and apparent pathological vein color changes appear on the eyeball. A diagnosis of disease of Zang and Fu is concurred". Wang Kentang (1549-1613), a Ming

Dynasty physician, *Guidelines in Syndrome Differentiation and Treatment, Volume 7, The Eye*.

During the Ming Dynasty, Hua Tuo's method was lost. His sayings though, inspired Professor Peng Jingshan. In 1970, Professor Jinshan began a clinical study in observing the eye to diagnose and treat disease based on these ancient records.

About the Inventor

Professor Peng Jingshan was born in Liaoning Province, China in 1909. At the age of fifteen, he began to study traditional Chinese medicine from many famous physicians. He diligently studied the classics, showing an excellent memory and outstanding comprehension. While he was studying acupuncture with Dr. Tang Yungun, he attained a firm foundation for practice by strengthening his fingers through exercise and also regulating Qi to them. In the early thirties he started his practice in Shenyang and achieved recognition immediately as a gifted practitioner. During this period he studied Western medicine to enhance his medical knowledge.

In the early fifties, he became a college teacher at the Chinese Medical University and started an acupuncture department in the clinics affiliated with the hospital. This was the first time acupuncture treatment was provided in an organized hospital setting, and this has since become the operating model throughout China. In 1950, Professor Peng wrote his first book *Simple Acupuncture Therapy* to help the beginning acupuncturists in Asia.

Now eighty-seven years old, he has taught at Liaoning College of Traditional Chinese Medicine from 1958 to present, and continues to work hard for the development of TCM. In his continuing career of more than sixty years, Professor Peng has written fourteen books, over 130 papers and received numerous awards. His most noted topic has been the invention of Ocular Acupuncture Therapy.

Professor Peng was the head of the Acupuncture Department and the vice-president of the college during the cultural revolution, and as a result, he was victimized. He became deaf due to beatings. In 1970, at age 61,

Professor Peng was of legal retirement age, but chose to return to the Acupuncture Department and resume work as a doctor. Due to his deafness, he faced many problems in his practice such as interpreting patients' complaints, voice and breath sounds, and cough and heartbeat. He was left with only two of the four TCM methods of diagnosis: observation and palpation. Professor Jinshan was fortunate enough to have excellent vision, therefore substituting sight for his loss of hearing.

When he reviewed Dr.Wang Kentang's writings about Hua Tuo's theory of eye diagnosis, he realized he was on the right path and began observing the eye for diagnostic purposes. In 1974 be experimented on 10,000 subjects using his eye diagnosis and then compared these findings with physicians' diagnoses using the four methods. The accuracy rate proved to be 90%.

In his first case, acute abdominal pain caused by a round worm in the gallbladder duct, he observed the eyes and realized the capillary branches of the gallbladder region of the right eye were extremely red, bright and enlarged. He inserted one needle in the gallbladder region of the right eye orbit. The severe pain was completely relieved fifteen minutes after the needle insertion. This amazing result encouraged him to try this technique on many difficult cases which had shown no improvement with herbs.

Hence, Ocular Acupuncture Therapy was born as another unique micro-acupuncture therapy. It was then introduced on different cases in the acupuncture department and, in 1982, was evaluated and approved as a new therapy by the government of Liaoning Province. In 1983, the media brought this new technique to all of China. The first nationwide seminar, held in Beijing in 1986, brought this new therapy even greater recognition in China. Professor Peng spoke in November of 1987 at the First World Conference on Acupuncture-Moxibustion, which was held in Beijing. One thousand five hundred delegates from fifty countries attended. Since then, this technique has gained worldwide recognition. Acupuncturists from many countries, including the United States of America, have come to the Liaoning College of Traditional Chinese Medicine to study under Professor Peng and his research department. His dedication and success in acupuncture has granted him the distinction of being one of the top four acupuncturists in China.

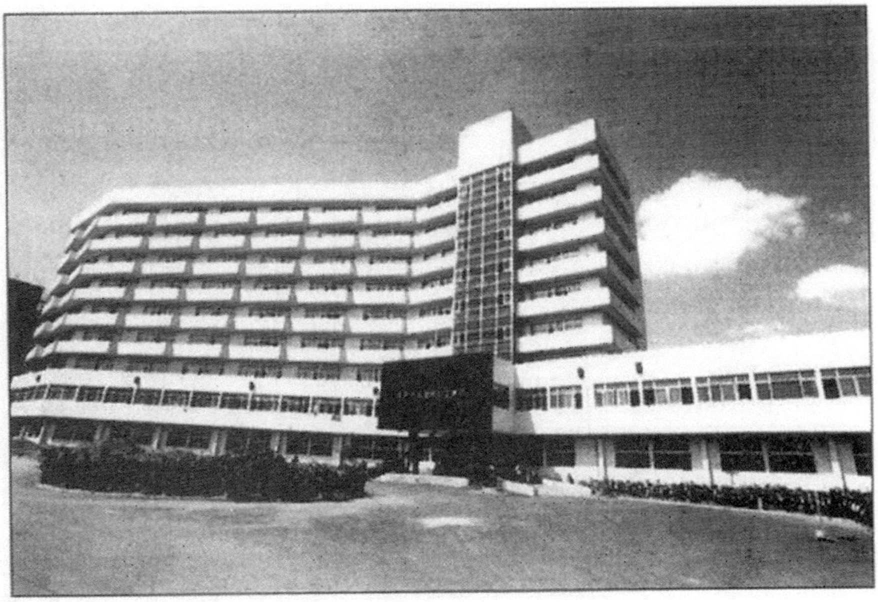

Figure 2 The Hospital of Liaoning College of TCM

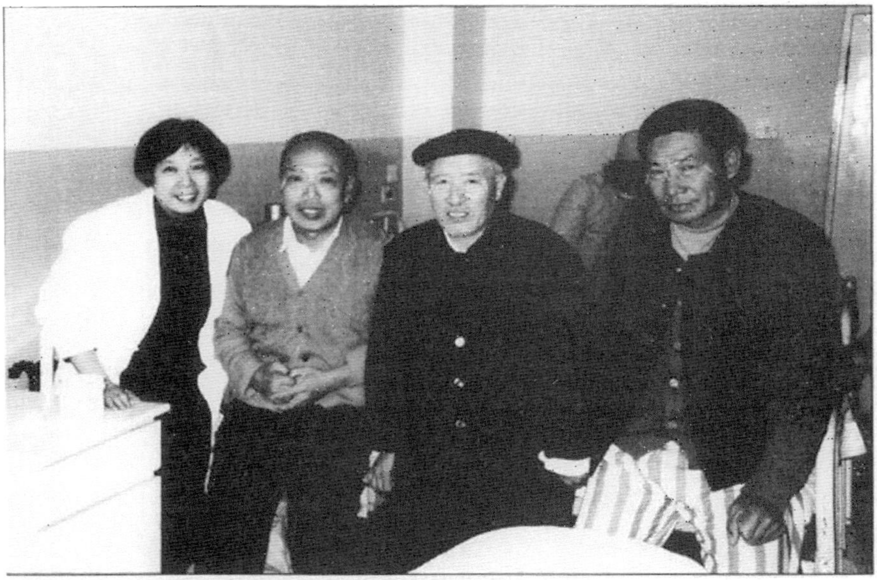

Figure 3 Dr. Chan with Stroke Patients at Liaoning College of Traditional Chinese Medicine in 1993

CHAPTER TWO

Relative Anatomy

For a deeper understanding of ocular diagnosis and periocular acupuncture and to avoid the possibility of accidents during treatments, the anatomy relative to periocular needling technique should be clear.

The Superficial Look and Skin of Palpebrae

The palpebrae, or eyelids, are divided into two parts: an upper and lower. The superior border of the upper eyelid is distinct where it meets the eyebrow at the orbit. However, this juncture or groove is not noticeable when the eye is open. The inferior border of the lower eyelid is not nearly as distinct in relation to the orbit due to layers of soft tissue. However, in older people, since the tissues surrounding the orbit may be less substantial, it is easy to find two distinct shadowy grooves where the skin crosses over the orbital bones. The free edge of the palpebra, where the eyelashes emerge, is called the palpebral margin. At the very edge of the palpebral margin is a thin gray line dividing the palpebra into an anterior portion and a posterior portion. The anterior portion includes skin, subcutaneous tissue and m. orbicularis oculi. The posterior portion includes the palpebral conjunctiva and tarsus (eyelid plate). The palpebra conjunctiva lines the inner surface of the eyelids and, doubling back over itself, passes from the eyelids onto the anterior surface of the eyeball. This portion is called the bulbar conjunctiva.

The skin of the eyelid is the thinnest skin on the body. It is very flexible and easy to stretch and therefore easy to wrinkle. Connective tissue is attached to the palpebral skin. Fatty tissue may also appear here on some people. Muscle tissues are located just beneath the level of the connective tissue. (Figure 4)

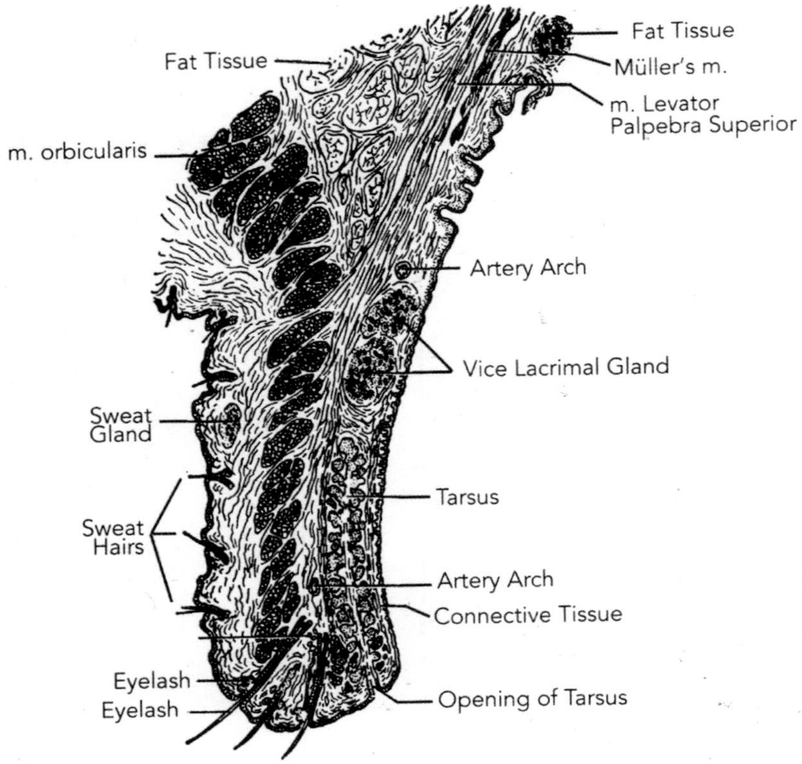

Figure 4 The Palpebra

The Muscles

M. orbicularis oculi

This is the main muscle of the palpebra. It is divided into three parts. The muscle on the outside lies around the orbit. Its fibers start from the inner canthus, encircle the orbit, and return to the inner canthus. Movements of this part of the muscle are voluntary. The upper and lower eyelids are closed tightly when this muscle is contracted. (Figure 5)

The central part of m. orbicularis oculi is at the third layer of the palpebra and is shaped like a half of an oval. Its fibers start at the inner canthus and end at the outer canthus. The movements of this part of the muscle is involuntary. Its movement may be slightly aided by closing the eyelids.

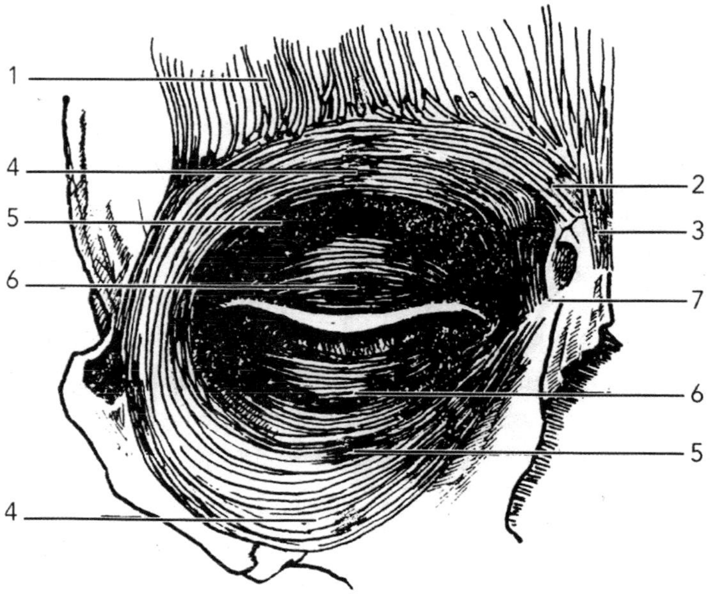

1. m. frontal
2. m. eyebrow motion
3. m. corrugator supercilii
4. m. orbicularis oculi around the orbit
5. m. orbicularis oculi the part between orbit and palpebra
6. m. orbicularis oculi on the front of palpebra
7. inner canthus

Figure 5 M. orbicularis oculi

A very small third part of the muscle lying by the tear sac is called m. Horner. Its function is to push the eyelid closer to the surface of the eyeball. The purpose of this is to drain tears through the lacrimal passage down to the tear sac. (Figure 5) The movement of the orbicular muscle is controlled by n. facial.

M. Müller

This is a piece of thin smooth muscle lying below the m. orbicularis oculi. It is controlled by the sympathetic nervous system. The eyelids open wider if its fibers are contracted. (Figure 4)

M. levator palpebra superior

A thin muscle which starts at the top of the m. rectus superior and ends at the upper eyelid as a piece of fascia, is controlled by n. oculomotorius. Its function is to raise the upper palpebra when contracting. (Figure 4)

The Sensory Nerve

The sensation of the palpebra is supplied by the first and second branches of the trigeminal nerve, which is the 5th cranial nerve.

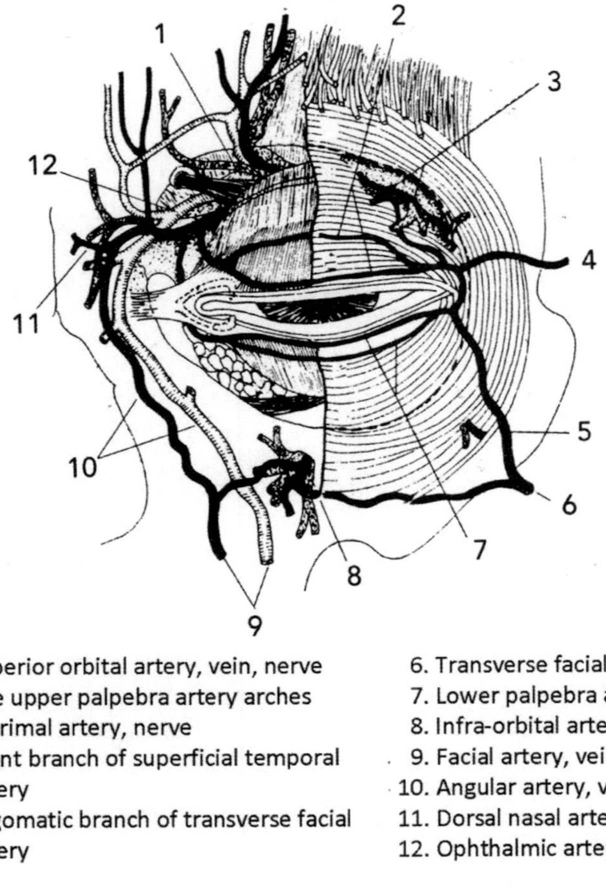

1. Superior orbital artery, vein, nerve
2. The upper palpebra artery arches
3. Lacrimal artery, nerve
4. Front branch of superficial temporal artery
5. Zygomatic branch of transverse facial artery
6. Transverse facial artery
7. Lower palpebra artery arch
8. Infra-orbital artery, nerve
9. Facial artery, vein
10. Angular artery, vein
11. Dorsal nasal artery
12. Ophthalmic artery

Figure 6 The Arterial Supply to Palpebra

The Circulation

The Arterial Supply to the Palpebra

The blood flow of the palpebra is supplied by the branches of the facial arterial system: the angular artery, the superficial temporal artery, and the infraorbital artery. The blood of this system originates from the external carotid artery and then connects to the branches of the ophthalmic artery, which is one of the larger branches from the internal carotid artery. At the deeper part of the palpebra, the network forms a palpebra arterial arch. (Figure 6)

The Arterial Supply to the Bulbar Conjunctiva

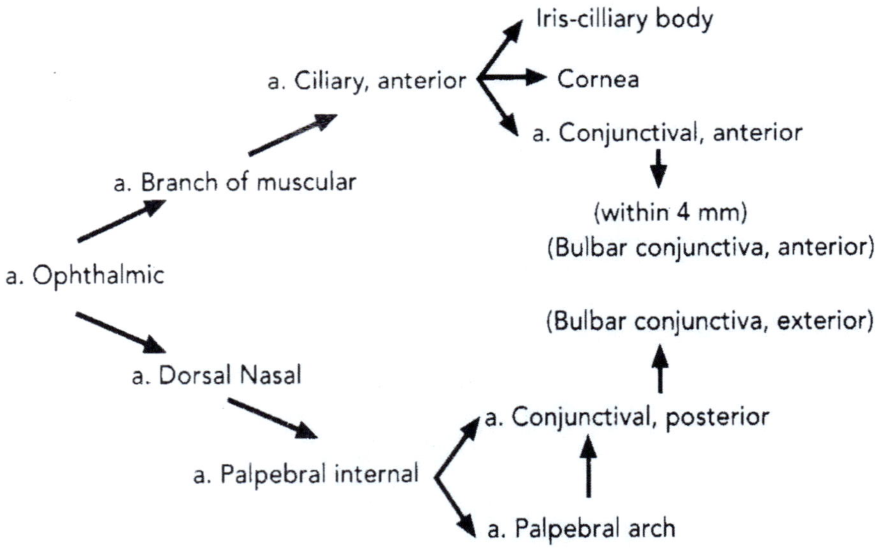

Figure 7 Arterial Supply to the Bulbar Conjunctiva

The blood is supplied from the ophthalmic artery to within 4 mm of the border in the area of the cornea. A branch from the ophthalmic artery forms the anterior ciliary artery which then branches to become the anterior conjunctival artery. (Figure 6) Clinically, when this area of the bulbar conjunctiva is inflamed, a serious condition may exist and the individual should be referred to a physician for further examination.

The blood in the external part of the bulbar conjunctiva comes from the palpebra internal artery. A branch of it forms the posterior conjunctival artery. These arteries stem from the dorsal nasal artery, which is itself another branch from the ophthalmic artery. These arterial branches form a capillary network in the external bulbar conjunctival area. Understanding the origins of the arterial flow within the bulbar conjunctiva can be an important key to aid in diagnosis. (Figure 8)

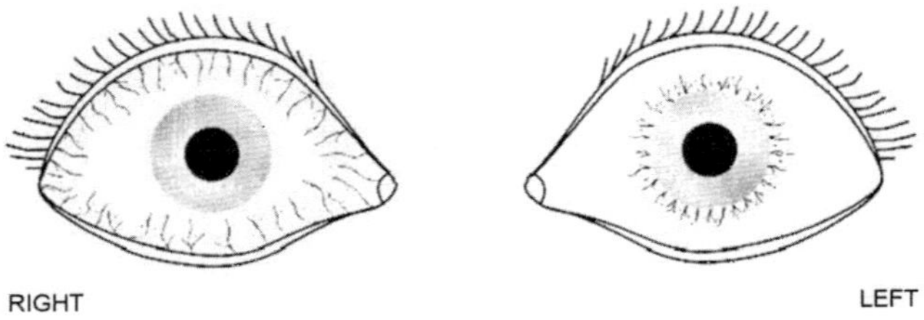

Figure 8 Conjunctival (R) vs. Ciliary Congestion (L)

Left Eye: To within 4 mm of the border of the cornea and anterior conjunctiva, the arterial blood is supplied by the a. anterior ciliary.

Right Eye: In the exterior conjunctiva, the arterial blood is supplied by the a. palpebral internal.

The Venous Collection

The venous collection routes are not as stable as the arterial supply to the bulbar conjunctiva so it can vary in different people. From the venous network there are two palpebra vein arches, one flowing directly to the v. angular while the other goes from the inner vein arch and then flows to the angular vein, then the facial vein, and finally the external jugular vein. The outer vein arch goes to the superior temporal vein, then flows to the external jugular vein. More venous blood is collected by the lacrimal vein, the ophthalmic vein, and then the internal jugular vein. The angular, facial, and ophthalmic veins are without valves on the interior walls of the vessels. Therefore blood could flow back into the cavernous sinus within the cranium. If there is any infection, it may result in a severe infection inside the cranium.

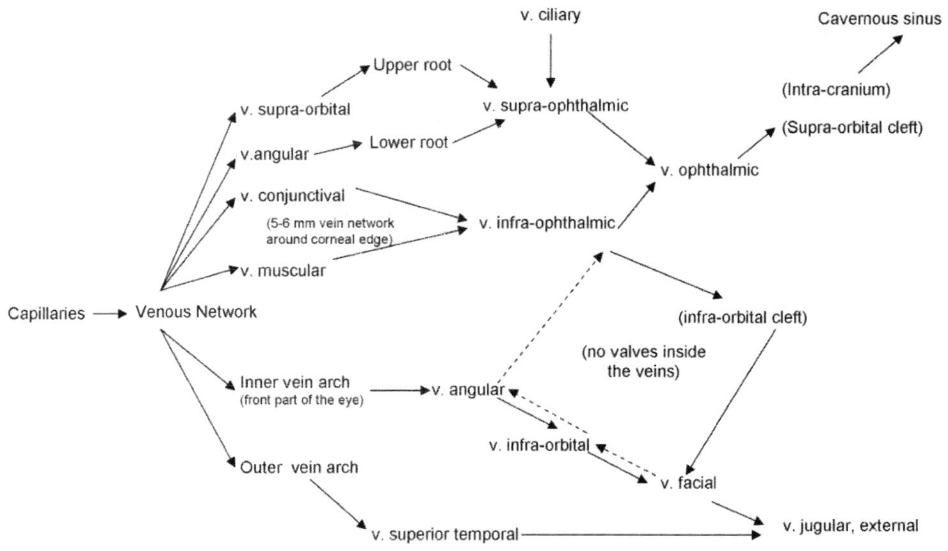

Figure 9 The Venous Collection to the Bulbar Conjunctiva

The Distribution of the Nerves and Arteries in the Deeper Layer of each Periocular Region

The following lists the nerves and arteries in the deeper layer of each of the periocular regions: (For the location of the eight periocular regions see Chapter Four)

1. **Region I:** Branches of the supraorbital nerve and arteries network; the branch of the frontal nerve.

2. **Region II**: Branches of the supraorbital nerve and arteries network; the branch of the lacrimal nerve.

3. **Region III**: Branches of the supraorbital nerve and lacrimal nerve; the lacrimal artery and the frontal branch of the superficial temporal artery; the network of the zygomatic orbital artery.

4. **Region IV**: Palpebral branch of the infraorbital nerve; the network of the infraorbital and the superficial temporal arteries.

5. **Region V**: Branch of the infrapalpebral of the infraorbital nerve; the infraorbital artery network.

6. **Region VI**: Branch of the infrapalpebral of the infraorbital nerve; the infraorbital artery.

7. **Region VII**: Branches of the infrapalpebral of the infraorbital nerve and the infratrochlear nerve; the arterial network for the angular artery and infraorbital artery.

8. **Region VIII**: Branches of the frontal nerve and the supratrochlear nerve; the arterial network for the supraorbital artery and the frontal artery.

The above anatomy of these regions was demonstrated by Professor Peng and the doctors of the Anatomy Department of Liaoning College of Traditional Chinese Medicine.

CHAPTER THREE

Theory

The Eye and Meridians

There are eight meridians which have a direct relationship with the eye. The Lung, Pericardium, Spleen, and Kidney channels do not. However, when looking at the internal and external relationships of the Lung and Large Intestine, Spleen and Stomach, Kidney and Bladder, and the Pericardium and Triple Warmers, then the twelve regular meridians all connect to the eye.

A. Meridians which begin from the eye and periocular region

1. The Stomach channel begins from the side of the nose intersecting the Bladder channel at B1 (Jingming). The first point of the Stomach channel, ST1 (Chengji), is located below the pupil right at the center of the margin of infraorbitalis. (Figure 10)
2. The Bladder channel starts from the inner canthus at B1 (Jingming). (Figure 11)
3. The Gallbladder channel begins from the outer canthus at GB1 (Tongziliao). (Figure 12)

B. Meridians which run through the eye and periocular region

1. The Heart channel has a branch of its main channel which separates in the Heart and ascends alongside the esophagus to the face and reaches the eye. (Figure 13)
2. The Liver channel has an internal course which runs upward across the diaphragm, the neck, posterior to the pharynx, and enters the nasopharynx before connecting to the eye. (Figure 14)

3. The Governing channel (Du Mai) runs between the two eyes and reaches the bridge of the nose, then ends at the midpoint between the inside of the upper lip and the gum. The origin of the third path is in common with that of the Bladder channel at the inner canthus of the eye. (Figure 15)

4. The Conception channel (Ren Mai) intersects the Stomach channel at ST1 (Chengji) below the orbit on the face. (Figure 16)

5. The Yang Linking channel (Yangwei Mai) intersects the Gallbladder channel, and one of its coalescent points at GB14 (Yangbai) on the forehead above the eye. (Figure 17)

6. The Yin Linking channel (Yinwei Mai) meets the Conception channel at the throat with the coalescent points Ren22 (Tiantu) and Ren23 (Lianquan). (Figure 17)

C. Meridians which end at the eye and periocular region

1. Large Intestine channel ends at the side of the nose and meets the Stomach channel. From there it connects with the eye. (Figure 18)

2. Triple Warmer (Sanjiao) channel has the last point, TW23 (Sizhukong), located at the lateral end of the eyebrow. A branch runs downward to the infraorbital region and intersects with the Small Intestine channel. (Figure 19)

3. Small Intestine channel has a branch which runs to the inner canthus where it meets the Bladder channel at B1 (Jingming). The other branch reaches the outer canthus where it meets the Gallbladder channel at GB1 (Tongziliao). (Figure 20)

4. Yang Heel channel (Yangqiao Mai) is an extra channel which enters the inner canthus at point B1 (Jingming) to communicate with the other extra channel Yin Heel (Yinqiao Mai). (Figure 21)

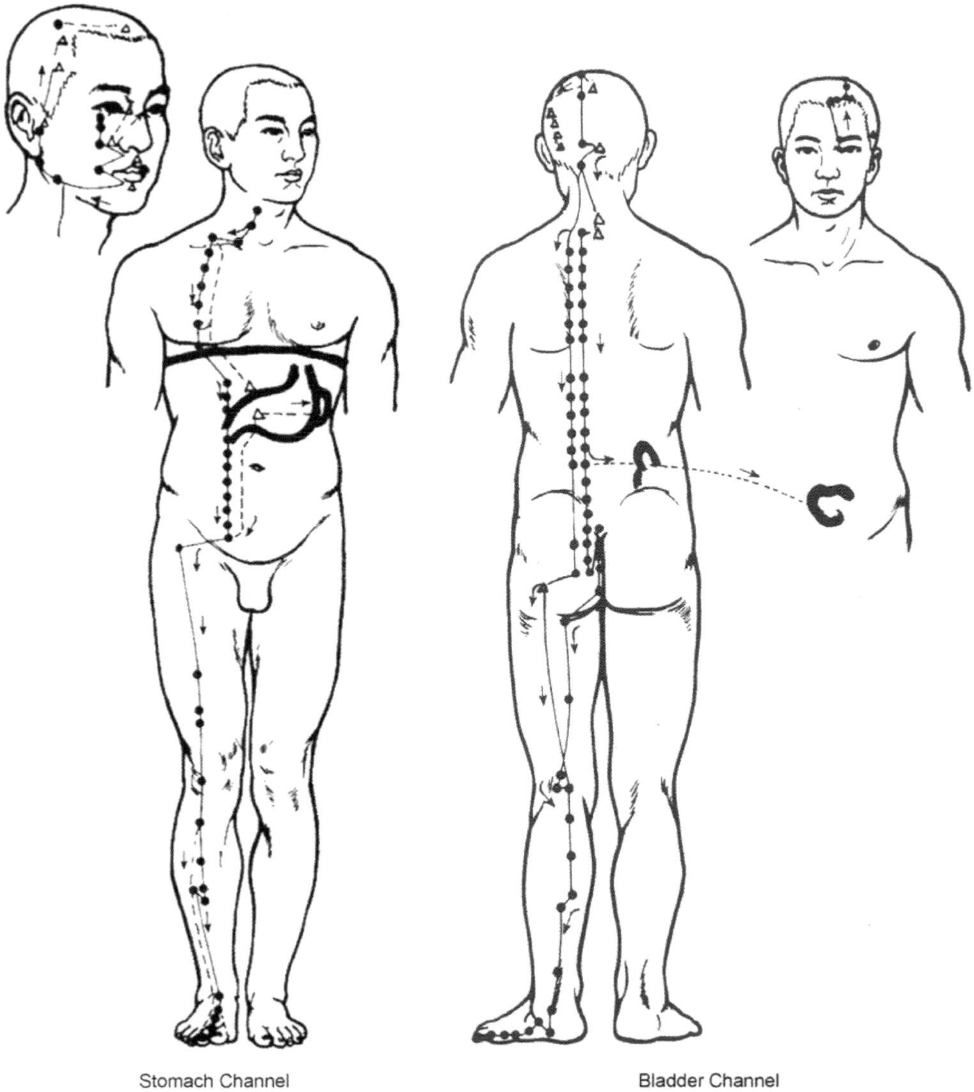

Figure 10 The Stomach Channel of Foot - Yangming

Figure 11 The Bladder Channel of the Foot - Taiyang

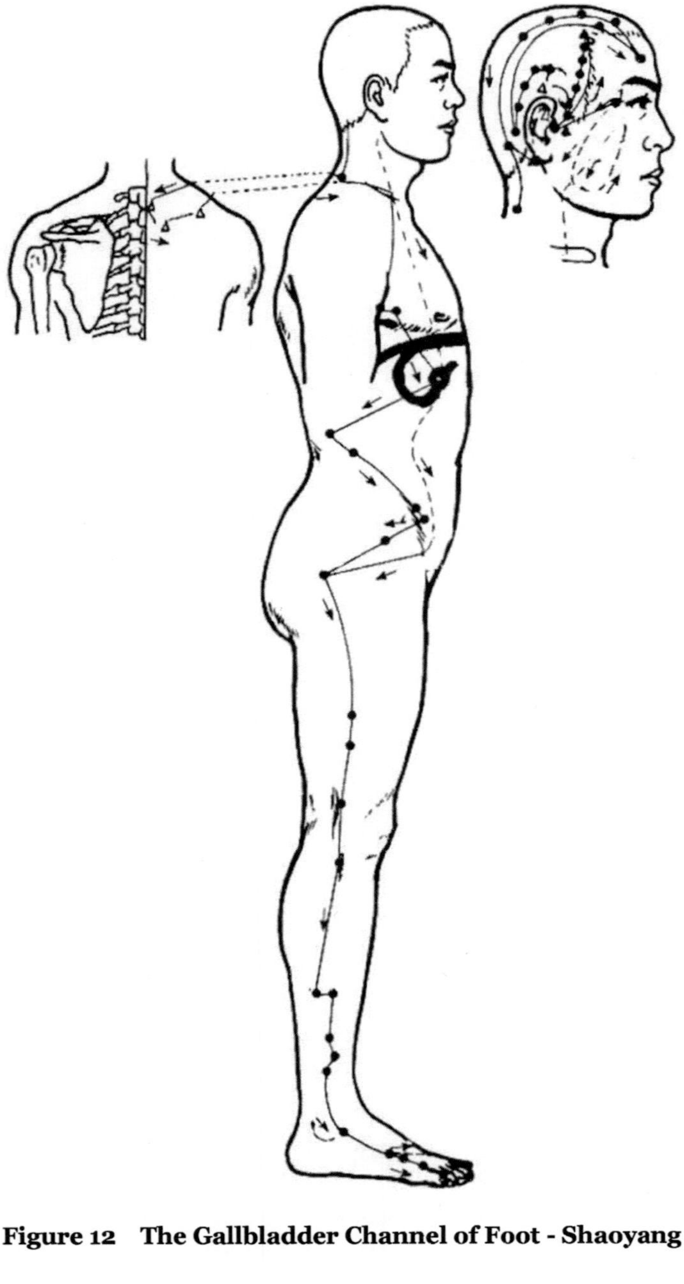

Figure 12 The Gallbladder Channel of Foot - Shaoyang

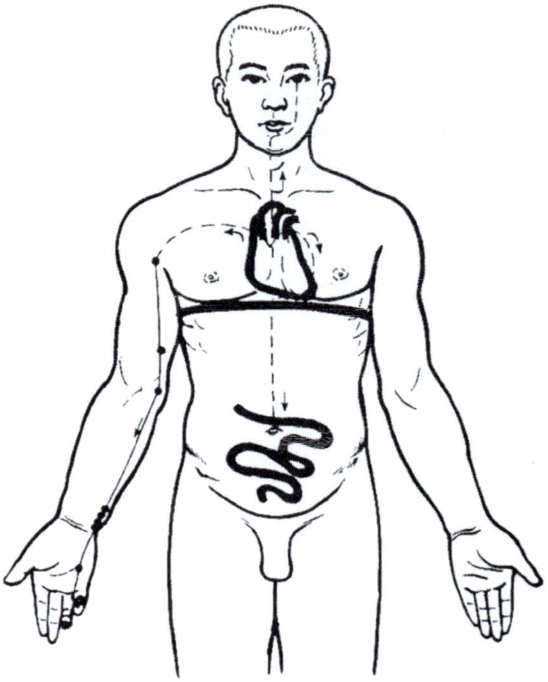

Heart Channel

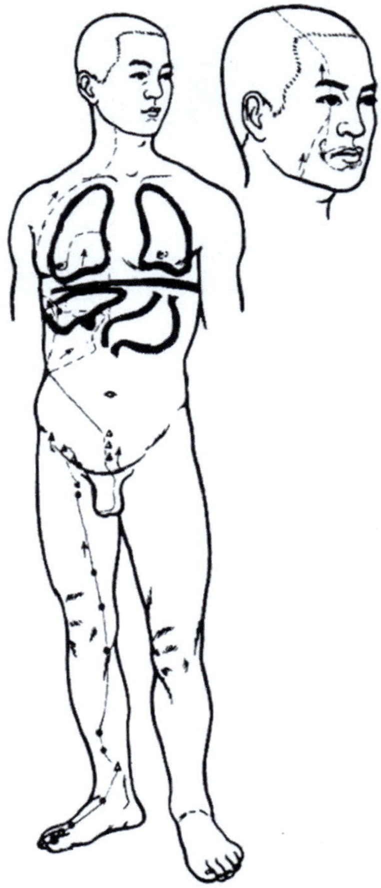

Liver Channel

Figure 13 The Heart Channel of the Hand - Shaoyang

Figure 14 The Liver Channel of Foot - Jueyin

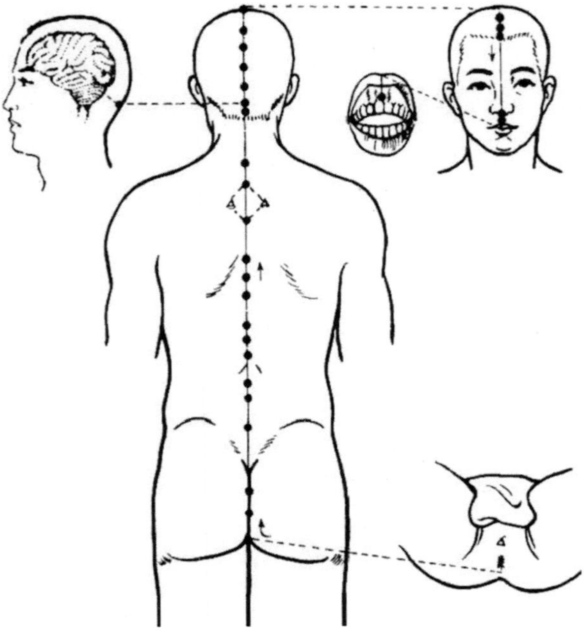

Figure 15 The Governing Vessel - Du Mai

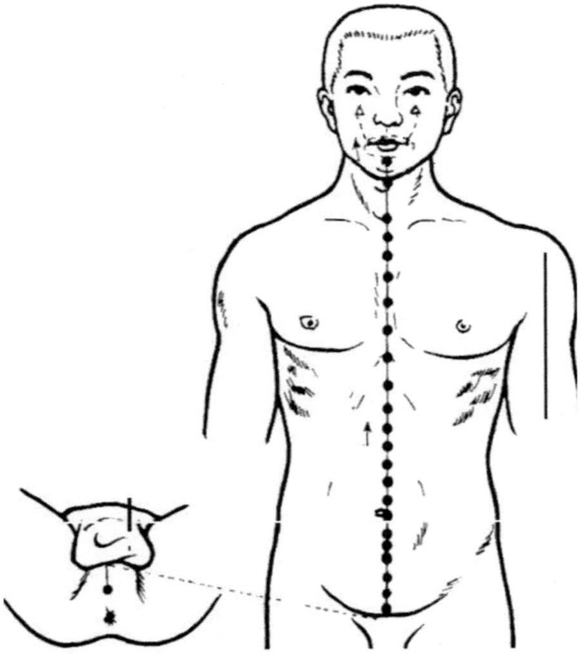

Figure 16 The Conception Channel - Ren Mai

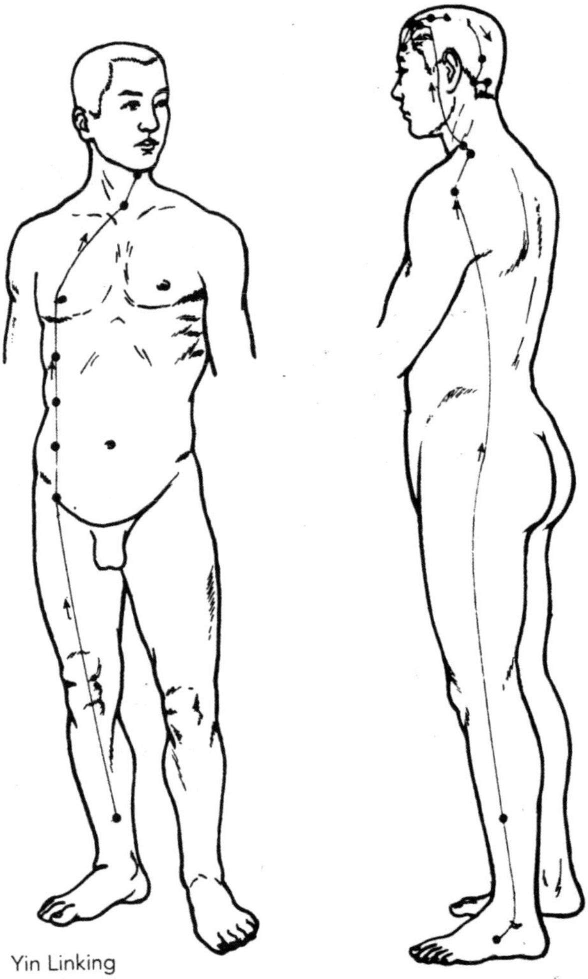

Figure 17 The Yin and Yang Linking Channels - Yin Wei Mai and Yan Wei Mai

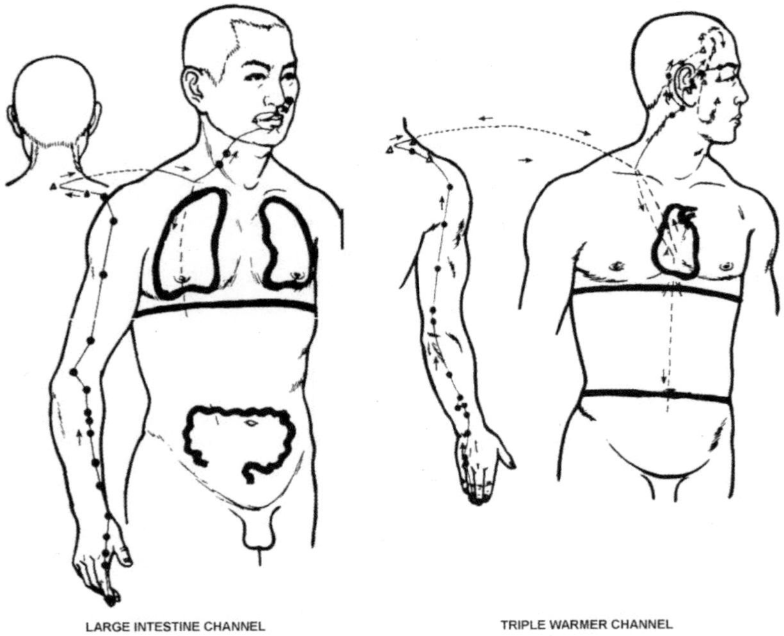

Figure 18 The Large Intestine Channel of Hand - Yangming

Figure 19 The Triple Warmer Channel of Hand - Shaoyang

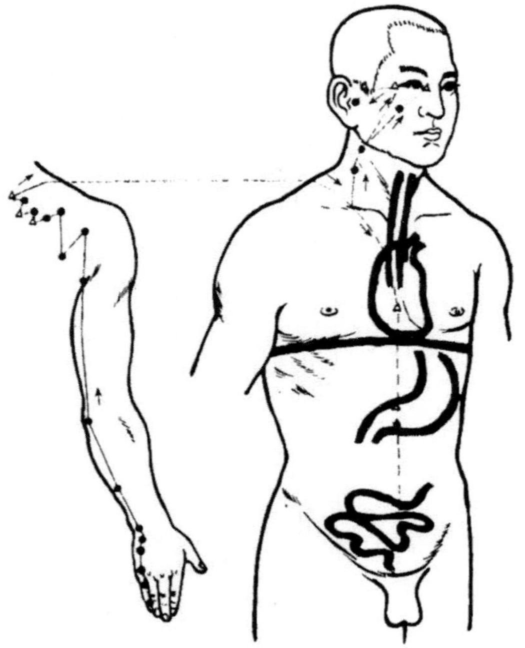

Figure 20 The Small Intestine Channel of Hand - Taiyang

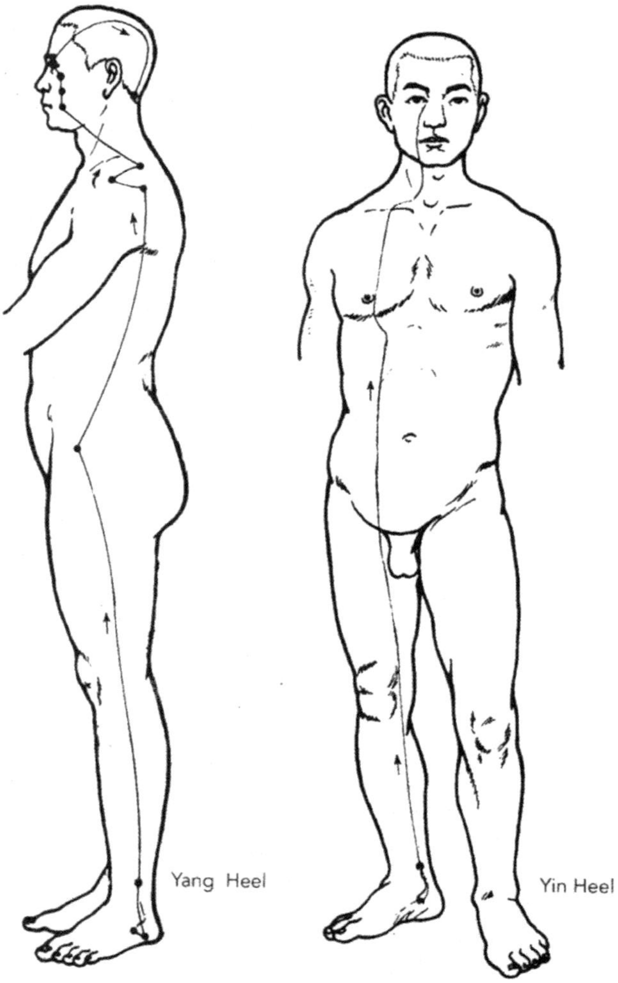

Figure 21 The Yang Heel and Yin Heel Channels - Yang Qiao Mai and Yin Qiao Mai

The Eye and Muscle Regions

The muscle regions originate from the extremities and ascend to the head and trunk but do not reach Zang-Fu organs. Similar to the twelve regular meridians, they are also divided into three hand Yin and three hand Yang, three foot Yin and three foot Yang. The muscle regions are distributed under the skin.

A. Muscle Region of the Bladder: One of its branches spreads around the eye and knots at the side lateral to the nose. (Figure 22)

B. Muscle Region of the Gallbladder: A sub-branch knots with the outer canthus. (Figure 23)

C. Muscle Region of the Stomach: A branch from the nose ascends to join the muscle region of the Bladder to form a muscle net around the lower region of the eye. (Figure 24)

D. Muscle Region of the Small Intestine: One of its branches runs upward to link with the outer canthus. (Figure 25)

E. Muscle Region of the Triple Warmer: A branch proceeds upward in front of the ear to the outer canthus. (Figure 26)

F. Muscle Region of the Large Intestine: A branch separates and connects at the side of the nose where it links with the muscle region of Stomach and Bladder. (Figure 27)

In conclusion, the relationship between the meridians and the muscle regions which nourish the eye are very close together and form a complete network for Qi and Blood flow to the eye.

The Eye and Organs (Zang-Fu)

The Heart and Small Intestine

The heart dominates the blood and vessels. All vessels belong to the eye. The blood in the vessels circulates throughout the whole body and flows to the eye, nourishing for clear vision.

One of the principle functions of the heart is associated with the spirit. Deficient Heart Qi shows a lack of vitality in a person's face and diminished light of spirit within the eye. The heart governs the mind and spirit and is the commander of the organs. It drives the Organ Qi to nourish the eye, hence, the vision, the expression, and all the activity of the eye is controlled by the heart.

Looking at the eye's spirit and expression is the first step of the Chinese diagnostic method. The internal - external relationship between the eye and small intestine is associated with Fire. The function of the small intestine influences the heart, then the eye. Heat in the small intestine would cause redness and pain in the eye.

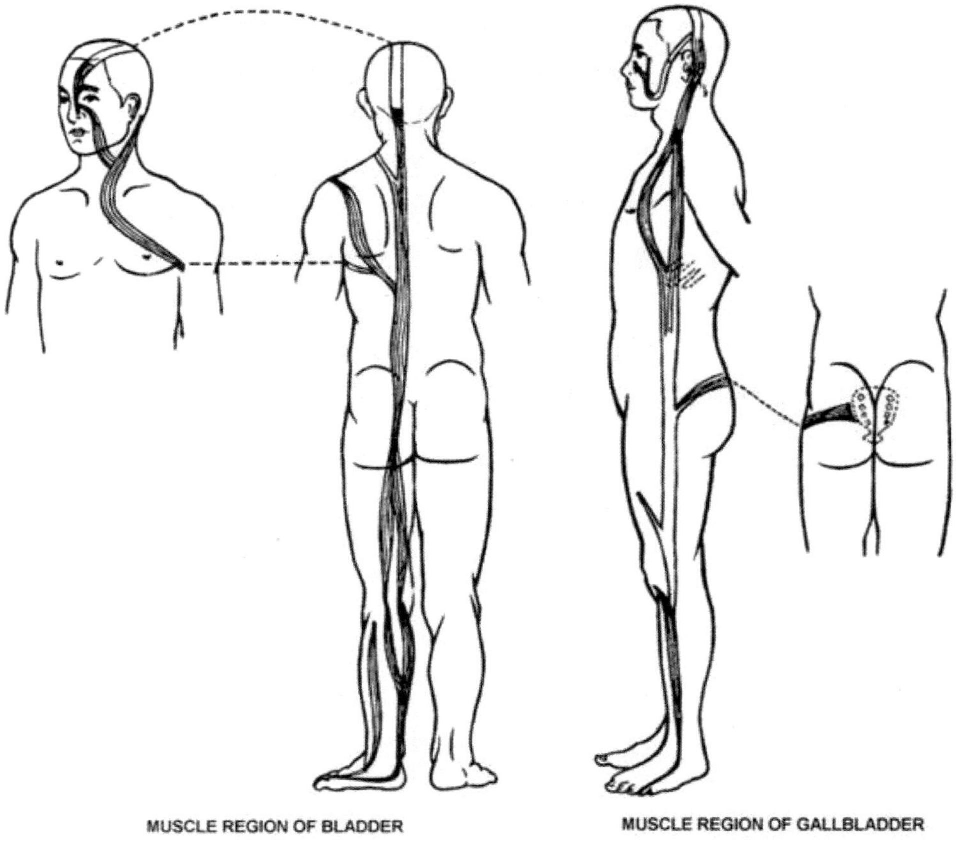

Figure 22 The Muscle Region of the Bladder
Figure 23 Muscle Region of Gallbladder

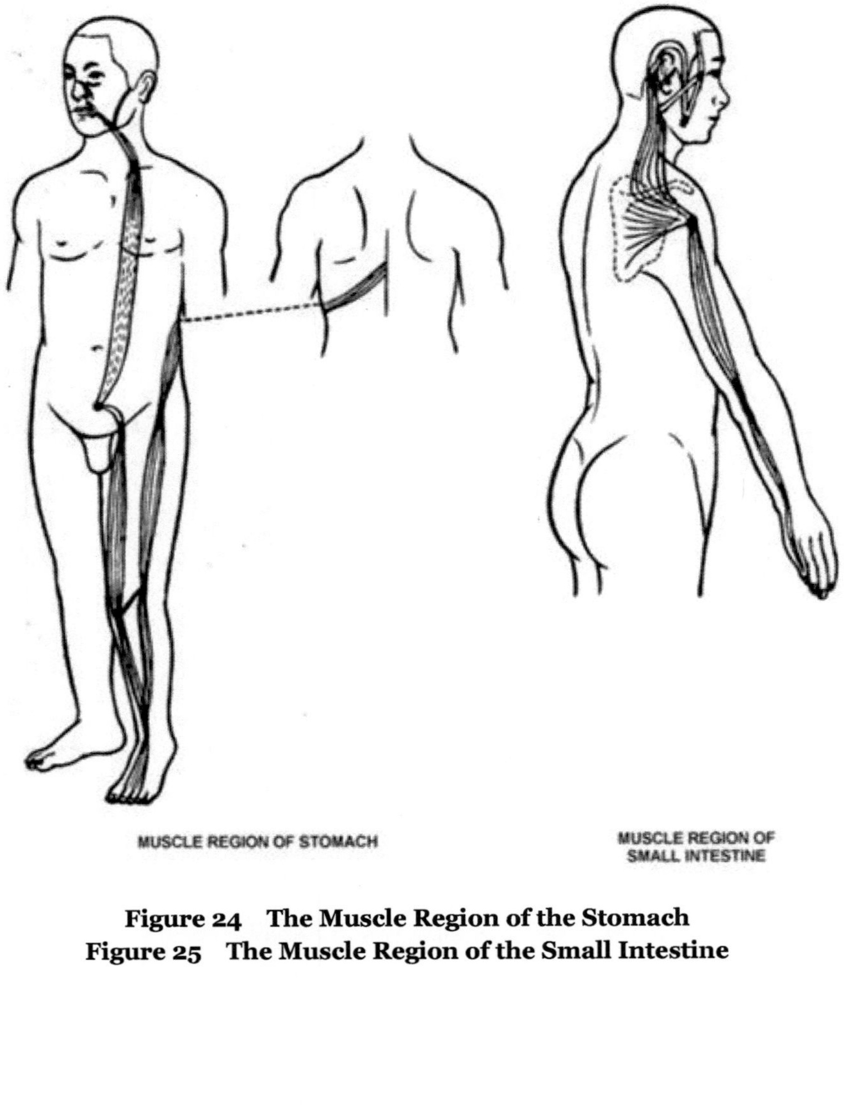

Figure 24 The Muscle Region of the Stomach
Figure 25 The Muscle Region of the Small Intestine

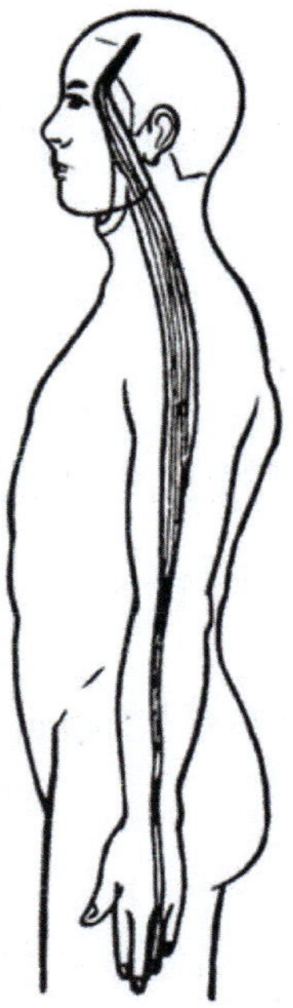

Figure 26 The Muscle Region of the Triple Warmer

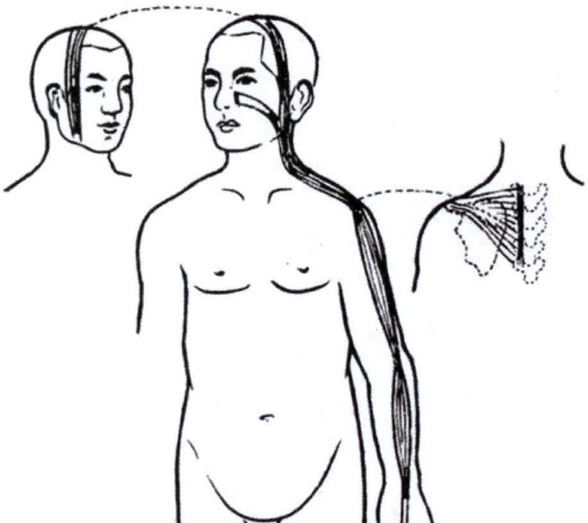

Figure 27 The Muscle Region of the Large Intestine

The Liver and Gallbladder

The liver's point of entry is the eye. It is the main organ affecting the eyes and vision. One of its most important functions is storage of blood. Its meridian ascends to connect with the eyes and whether the liver function is normal or not often reflects in the eyes. For example: deficiency of Liver Yin and Blood may lead to dryness of the eyes, blurred vision and even night blindness. When Deficient Liver Yin reaches a critical degree, the condition changes to rising Liver Yang or even Liver Fire, or Wind Heat. Such conditions of Heat in the Liver may occur causing irritation, redness, swelling and pain to the eye.

The balanced quality of Liver Qi is flowing and free and also reflects a state of harmony. Stagnation of Liver Qi would cause the eyes to have trouble seeing color or may even cause sudden blindness.

Dampness and Heat can affect the liver and gallbladder and cause a disorder disturbing the flow of bile. This in turn can produce a yellowing of both the skin and the eyes.

The Spleen and Stomach

The spleen is the principal organ of digestion. The transportation and transformation function of Spleen Qi should be ascending. When the spleen is weak, the body is unable to utilize the nourishment in food. The Spleen Qi is not strong enough to ascend, or indeed may sink, thereby causing vertigo, blurred vision, prolapse of various internal organs and diarrhea. Hence, the spleen is also closely related to the eye.

Deficient Spleen Qi would result in the loss of ability to govern the Blood. Blood would then not stay within the vessels and a hemorrhage might appear in the eye.

Based on the Five Wheels theory, the upper eyelid is associated with the spleen, and the lower eyelid corresponds to the stomach. Dampness in the spleen and stomach would show puffiness in the palpebrae.

The stomach couples with the spleen in both the internal - external and Yin and Yang relationships. It works together with the spleen for the digestive process.

The Kidney and Bladder

The kidneys form the Source Qi and store the Essence and are responsible for growth and development. The Essence creates the Marrow. The brain is the Sea of Marrow. The eye, through the nervous system, connects with the brain. When people are born with a lack of congenital essential substance, or have insufficient care after birth, the Source Qi is weak, which may contribute to eye diseases.

The kidney is said to be the "House of Water and Fire". Kidney Yin and Kidney Yang both restrict and promote each other in the human body to maintain balance. If either one fails, then there is created an imbalance between Yin and Yang. This may show as Water Deficiency or Fire Excess. These conditions would cause blurred vision or other discomfort in the eye. Deficient Kidney Yin can cause dark circles around the eye, especially under the eye.

The bladder transforms fluid into urine and excretes it from the body. When disorders appear, there is fluid retention which may result in swelling eyelids.

Lung and Large Intestine

The conjunctiva, a mucous membrane covering the anterior white part of the eye, is associated with the lung. It depends on the Lung Qi to form and maintain its function. Rebellious Lung Qi (coughing) might result in eye redness, or even appear as a hemorrhage of the conjunctiva.

The lungs govern Qi. A person with sufficient Qi shows a strong spirit and brightness in the eyes. The pupil contracts and stretches smoothly and actively. Weakness of Lung Qi may cause blurred vision. Collapsed of Lung Qi shows with a dilation of the pupil.

The internal - external relationship between the lung and large intestine results in the lungs moving the clear air into the body while the large intestine extracts water from the waste material and sends it on to the bladder, then excreting the solid material as stool. If the transportation of the large intestine is weak, then Heat will accumulate causing Fire to rise up with resulting painful and red eyes.

The Five Phases and Five Wheels

The ancient Chinese used another set of concepts in their attempt to understand the world. The Five Phases were regarded as five properties inherent in all things. They are Wood, Fire, Earth, Metal and Water. The Five Wheels theory is the application of the Five Phases to the eye. The purpose is to define the anatomy and physiology of different parts of the eye. The five anatomical parts are:

A. The Palpebrae: Muscle Wheel; spleen and Earth (the chief of the Five Phases); a yellowish color and the palpebrae opening and closing freely indicates health.

B. The Conjunctiva (White Eye): Qi Wheel; lung and Metal; a white color and moisture to the eye is healthy.

C. The Canthus: Blood Wheel; heart and Fire; the canthus should be red in color.

D. The Dark Eye: Wind Wheel; liver and Wood; green is the color to look for.

E. The Pupil: Water Wheel; kidney and Water; the color is black and clear.

The Five Wheels of the eye are associated with five organs. The disorders of the organs will reflect to the corresponding locations of the eye for diagnosis, prevention and treatment.

The Eight Diagrams (Bagua) and Eight Octants (Baguo)

The ancient Chinese physicians applied the Five Phases and Eight Octants theory to the eye. This theory was well developed during the thirteenth century. Many physicians had several different opinions about the Eight Octants and definitions and positions were unclear for a long period of time until the Chinese Ophthalmologist Fu Yunke (Fu Ren Yu) wrote a precious book on ophthalmology, *Shen Shi Yao Han*. He drew the eight positions on the eye to match with the Eight Octants (Baguo).

This book was written in the year 1644 and had seven volumes, listing one hundred and eight kinds of eye diseases and treatments. The Eight Octants

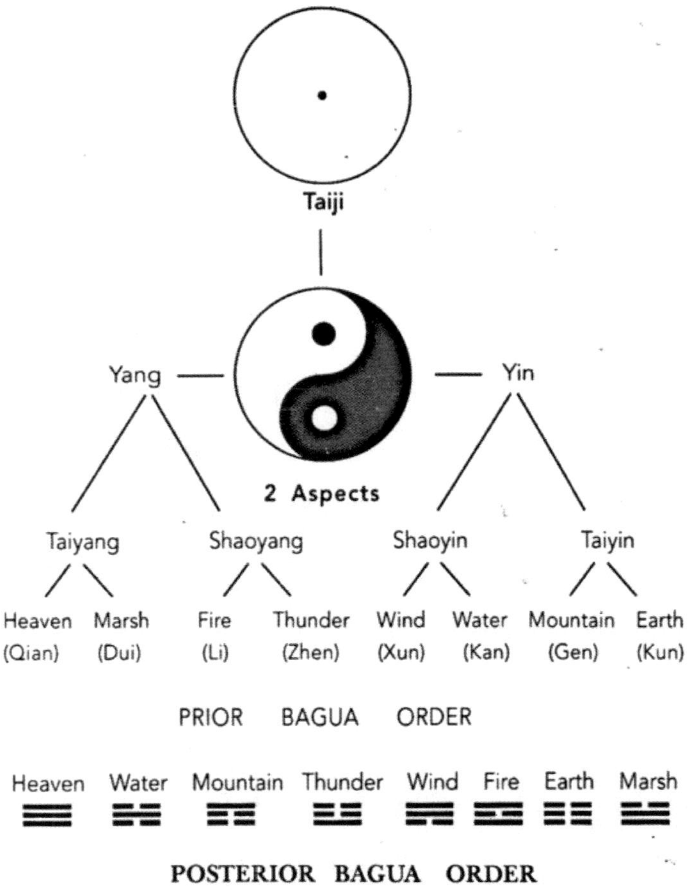

Figure 28 The Taiji Posterior Bagua

were given the name "Guo", which means "the walls of a city for protecting the place which is within the walls". The names of the Eight Octants were adopted from eight diagrams (Bagua Trigrams).

Professor Peng used his study of the Eight Diagrams and Eight Octants relating to the white of the eye in his theory of Ocular Acupuncture Therapy, in accordance with the ancient *Book of Changes* (*I Ching*). The Eight Diagrams originated from "Taiji", which was the beginning of all things. Next, two aspects, Yin and Yang were developed; then Four Diagrams appeared. The Four Diagrams became the Eight Diagrams which are represented by two symbols "— —" and "—". Historically, there are two kinds of Bagua, the anterior and the posterior. He thought the posterior Bagua more suitable to the eye. The order is: Qian (Heaven), Kan (Water), Gen (Mountain), Zhen (Thunder), Xun (Wind), Li (Fire), Kun (Earth), and Dui (Marsh). The eight regions on the bulbar conjuctiva are the Eight Octants of TCM ophthalmology based on the Eight Diagrams. (Figure 31)

Chinese physicians used the Eight Octants to match the Eight Diagrams. Qi and Blood flow in the meridians and collaterals, connecting the brain to organs that nourish the eye. The Octants have their own way for circulating the Qi and Blood to and from the eye.

The following are referenced to Figure 31, using the left eye.

A. Heaven (Qian): It is located at the north-northwest and is associated with the lung. It also corresponds to the large intestine. The lung accepts the fresh air and the large intestine excretes the wastes. Its function is to transport and has been given the name "Transmission Guo".

B. Water (Kan): It is located at the north-northeast and is associated with the kidney. It corresponds also to the urinary bladder. Because the kidney is related to water and transfers fluid, it has been given the name "Fluid Guo".

C. Mountain (Gen): It is located at the east-northeast and is associated with Mingmen. It corresponds to the Upper Warmer. It moves Qi throughout the whole body and has been given the name "Perineum Guo".

D. Thunder (Zhen): It is located at the east-southeast and is associated with the liver. It corresponds also to the gallbladder. Its function is to clean up toxins and has been given the name "Purity Guo".

E. Wind (Xun): It is located at the south-southeast and is associated with the Liver as well as the Middle Warmer. The Blood flows from the liver vessels to the Middle Warmer providing nourishment and has been given the name "Nourishing Guo".

F. Fire (Li): It is located at the south-southwest and is associated with the heart. It also corresponds to the small intestine. Because it is full of Yang, it has been given the name "Uterine Yang".

G. Earth (Kun): It is located at the west-southwest and is associated with the spleen and also corresponds to the stomach. Its function is to govern the food which supports the body and has been given the name "Foodstuff Guo".

H. Marsh (Dui): It is located at the west-northwest and is associated with the kidney as well as the lower warmer. Its function is to control the Yin Essence for growth and has been given the Name "Guanquan Guo".

CHAPTER FOUR

Location

To apply the location of the Eight Octants in clinical practice, ask the patient to lie in a supine position with the head north and the feet south. Using the face of a clock as an analogy, the first region is at 10:30 - 12:00, and is the direction of the Qian Diagram situated on the north-northwest of the individual's left eye. Because the left eye belongs to Yang, the following seven regions are counted clockwise for location.

The right eye belongs to Yin, and so the order is reversed and counted counter-clockwise. Professor Peng's first design on the right eye was to reverse the left eye to an upside down position. This position was changed in 1992 to what is seen in Figure 31.

Have the patient look straight ahead. The ocuzones are constructed by first drawing a horizontal line through the two canthi and a vertical line through the center of the pupil. The four resulting sections are bisected equally to form eight regions. Next, divide the five regions I, II, IV, VI, and VII evenly in two. As a result, the original eight regions have now become 13 ocuzones.

The Thirteen Ocuzones

Thirteen ocuzones make up the Eight Octants of the white of the eye. Containing one Zang and one Fu are five Octants: I, II, IV, VI, and VII. The following organ pairs are located in each of the respective Octants: I-Lung and Large Intestine, II-Kidney and Urinary Bladder, IV-Liver and Gallbladder, VI-Heart and Small Intestine and VII Spleen and Stomach. One of each of these pairs is located in half of each of their respective Octants. Occupying a whole region, are the octants III, V, and VIII, which consist of the Upper Warmer, Middle Warmer and Lower Warmer. (Figure 29)

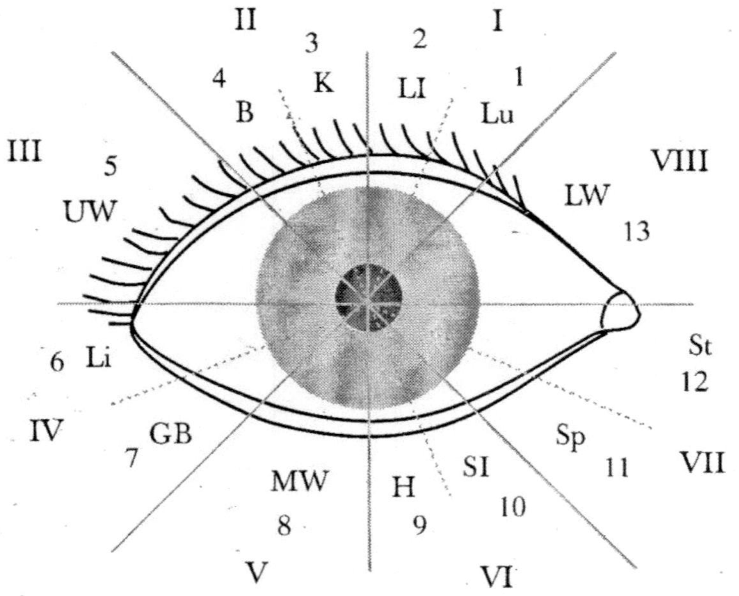

Figure 29 Ocuzones of the Right Eye

Note: The 13 ocuzones associated with the eyeball itself are used for diagnostic purposes only, as discussed in Chapter Five. The eyeball itself is never needled. The extension of the 13 ocuzones into the periocular regions is where actual needling takes place, as described in Chapters Six and Seven.

Triple Warmer Theory

The Triple Warmer (Sanjiao) vitalizes and coordinates all the body's functions. There are three sections of the Triple Warmer: Upper Warmer, Middle Warmer and Lower Warmer.

Miraculous Pivot says, "The Upper Warmer resembles the movement of fog; Middle Warmer absorbs and transfers; and the Lower Warmer acts as drainage for the excretory system". *Classical Medical Questions* writes, "Triple Warmer has a title but no form". Professor Peng points out that on the ocular region, the Triple Warmer should be interpreted in an expanded sense only. The Upper Warmer is located in the area above the diaphragm and contains the chest, upper back, organs, head, neck, and upper extremities. The Middle Warmer is the area located between the diaphragm and umbilicus and contains the upper and middle abdomen and organs. The Lower Warmer is the area located below the umbilicus and includes the lower abdomen and its organs, lumbar region and the lower extremities. Use boundaries to define areas which will aid in the discernment of clinical symptoms for ocular diagnosis and periocular needling. (Figure 30)

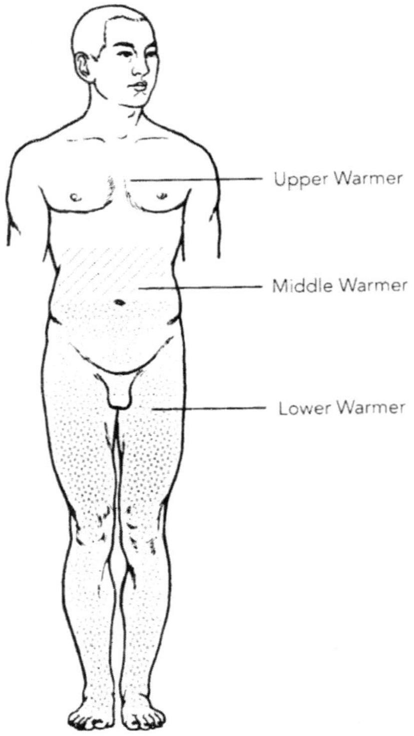

Figure 30 Triple Warmer in Ocular Diagnosis

Based on these boundaries, the Triple Warmer in this micro-acupuncture system treats all disorders. The Upper Warmer treats problems of the chest, including the heart, lungs, ribs, esophagus, trachea, head, neck, the five sense organs and the upper extremities. The Middle Warmer treats disorders of the lumbar, epigastrium, stomach, spleen, liver, gallbladder, pancreas and small intestine. The Lower Warmer is used for all illnesses of the lumbosacral region, pelvic cavity, buttocks, urogenital problems, small intestine, large intestine, colon, rectum, anus and lower extremities.

The Location

There are two kinds of ocuzones in the periocular region: intraorbital and extraorbital. The extraorbital zones are commonly used, and lie along the orbit of the eye, 5 mm distance from the edge. The four ocular regions above the eyeball are situated on the orbital margin along the lower line of the eyebrow. The four regions under the eyeball extend 2 mm below the infraorbital margin. The three single organ ocuzones are the III, V, and VIII regions and correspond to the Upper, Middle and Lower Warmers respectively. The other five regions are numbered I, II, IV, VI and VII and have two zones in each region: Lung and Large Intestine; Kidney and Urinary Bladder; Liver and Gallbladder; Heart and Small Intestine; Spleen and Stomach. Thus there are a total of thirteen periocular ocuzones. (Table 1)

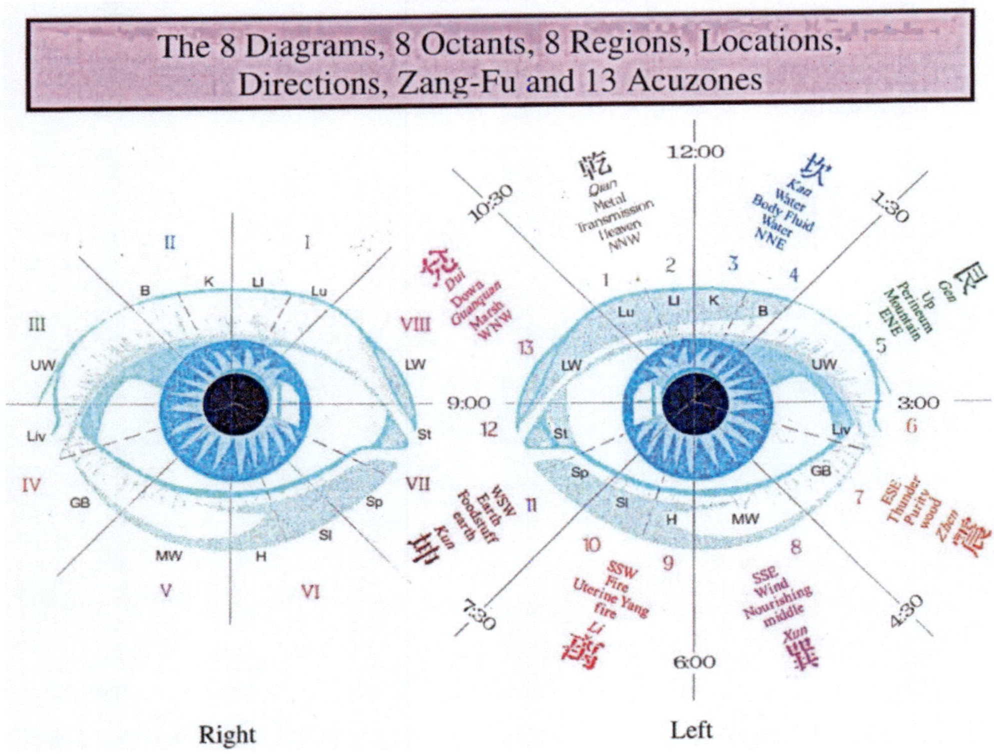

Figure 31 Location of Eight Regions, Eight Octants and 13 Ocuzones of the Individual's Left and Right Eyes

TABLE OF EIGHT REGIONS (Clock position, Direction, Name, Phenomena of Bagua, Symbol, Name & Function of Baguo, Acuzone, and Zang Fu)							
Region	**Clock Position**	**Direction**	**Bagua-Diagram Phenomena**	**Symbol**	**Baguo-Octant Function**	**Acu-zones**	**Zang-Fu Organs**
I	10:30 – 12:00	NNW	乾 *Qian* - Heaven	☰	Transmission	1	Lung
						2	Large Intestine
II	12:00 – 1:30	NNE	坎 *Kan* - Water	☵	Body Fluid	3	Kidney
						4	Bladder
III	1:30 – 3:00	ENE	艮 *Gen* - Mountain	☶	Perineum	5	Upper-Warmer
IV	3:00 – 4:30	ESE	震 *Zhen* - Thunder	☳	Purity	6	Liver
						7	Gall Bladder
V	4:30 – 6:00	SSE	巽 *Xun* - Wind	☴	Nourishing	8	Middle-Warmer
VI	6:00 – 7:30	SSW	离 *Li* - Fire	☲	Uterine Yang	9	Heart
						10	Small Intestine
VII	7:30 – 9:00	WSW	坤 *Kun* - Earth	☷	Foodstuff	11	Spleen
						12	Stomach
VIII	9:00 – 10:30	WNW	兑 *Dui* - Marsh	☱	*Guanquan*	13	Lower-Warmer

Table 1 Eight Regions

According to Professor Peng's explanation, these thirteen periocular ocuzones are not in common with the points located on the twelve regular channels and other extra points.. These are B1 (Jingming), B2 (Zanzhu), ST1 (Chengqi), ST2 (Sibai), GB1 (Tongziliao), GB14 (Yangbai), TW23 (Sizhukong). Extra points include Shangjingming, Xiajingming, Yuyao, Qiuhou. The thirteen ocuzones are found based on the Eight Diagram and Peng's experience, but the above mentioned points are located by the Channel Theory. (Figure 32)

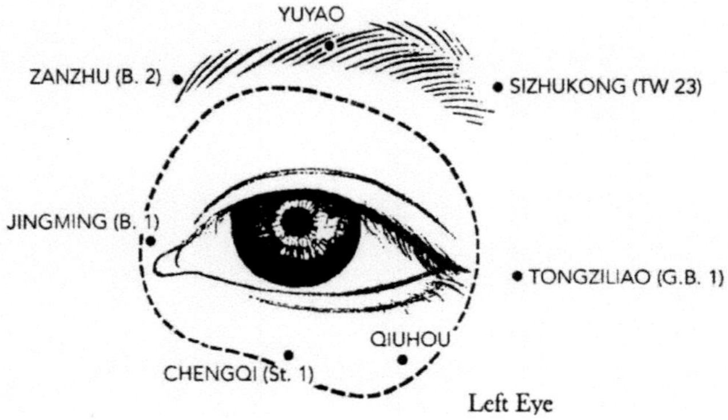

Figure 32 Points of 12 Regular Channels and Extra Points

CHAPTER FIVE

Disease Recognition

Through clinical practice and observation of the eye, Professor Peng developed a set of methods for recognizing a patient's disease.

Pathological Variances in the Capillary Branches of the Bulbar Conjunctiva

A. Broad stalks: observed in stubborn cases. (Figure 33)

B. Abnormally swollen, enlarged, prolonged and twisted: ill due to excess. (Figure 34)

C. Branches beyond ocuzone boundaries: illness is in more than one organ. (Figure 35)

D. Divided into branches: located usually under the pupil, variable illness easily changes to different kinds of symptoms. (Figure 36)

E. Capillaries standing out or raising up as a line of protrusion: illness is located in six Fu organs. (Figure 37 and 38)

F. Diamond-like shape: indicates illness with complicated symptoms. (Figure 39)

G. Indistinct region: usually observed in the Liver - Gallbladder divisions, symptoms of tension, stress and depression. (Figure 40)

H. Projecting as a dewdrop: if it shows on the Stomach and/or Intestine regions, points to parasitic infection; if it appears in other regions may be blood stagnation. (Figure 41)

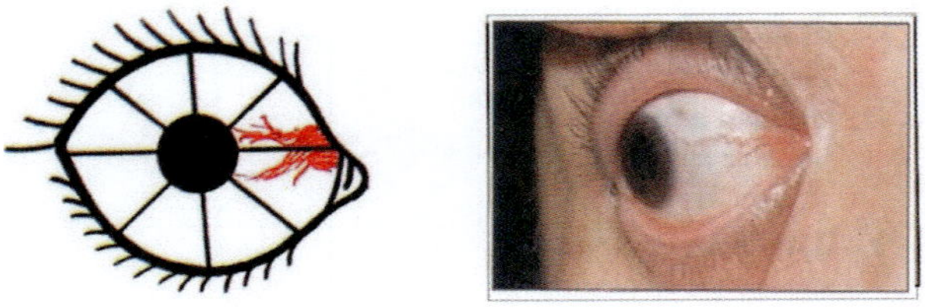

Figure 33 Broad Stalk, Enlarged and Prolonged

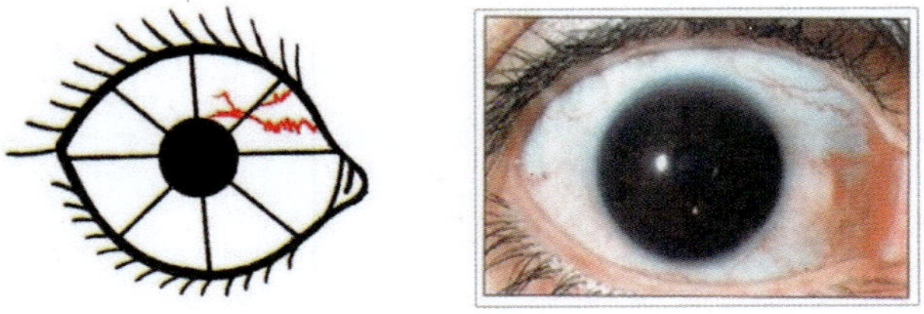

Figure 34 Abnormally Twisted

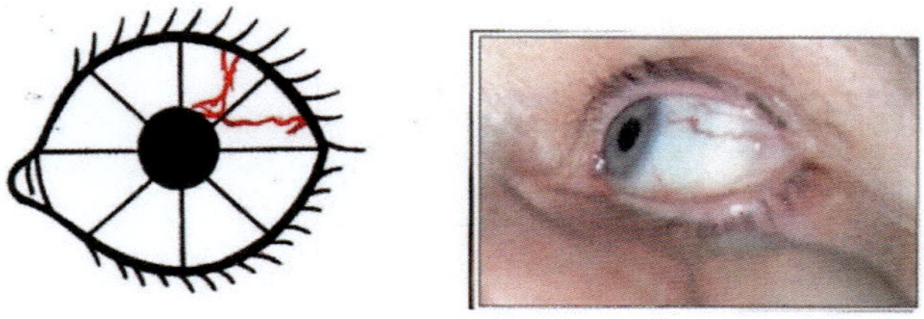

Figure 35 Branches Beyond Ocuzone Boundaries

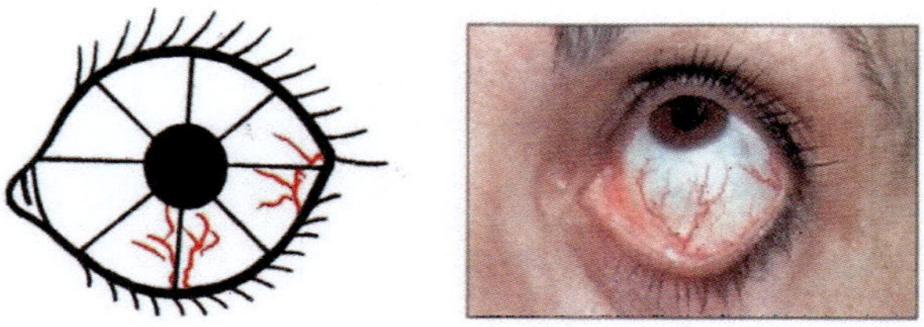

Figure 36 Divided into Branches

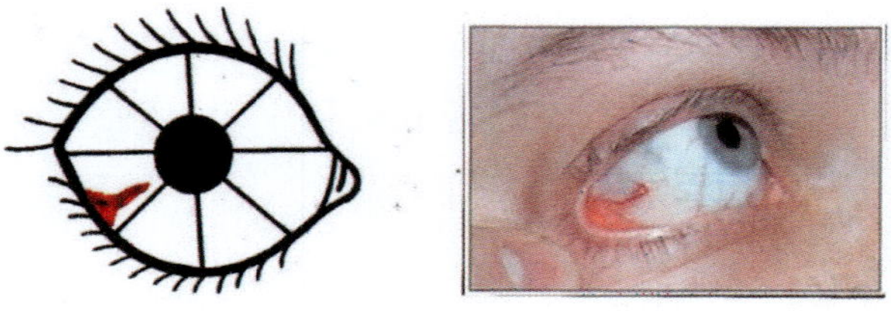

Figure 37 Capillaries Standing Out

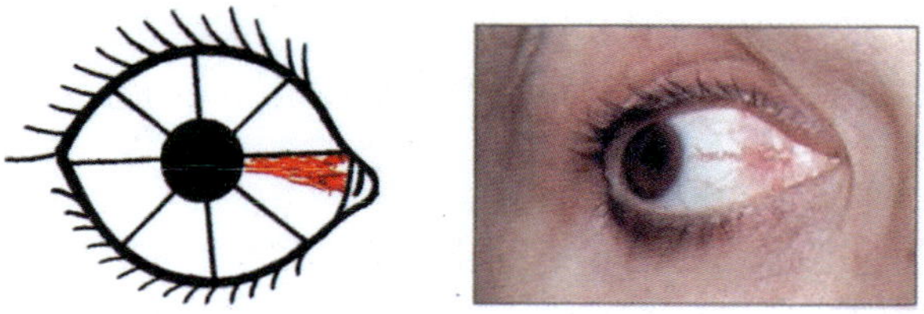

Figure 38 Raising Up as a Line of Protrusion

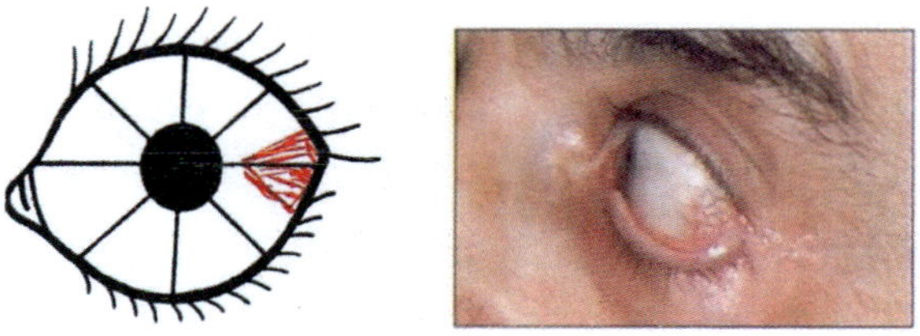

Figure 39 Diamond-Like Shape

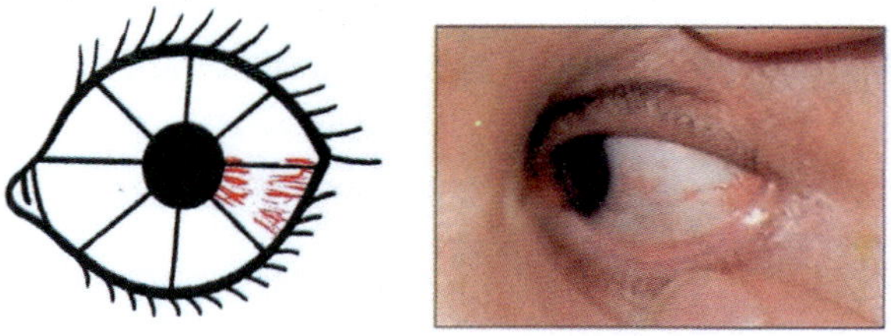

Figure 40 Indistinct Region

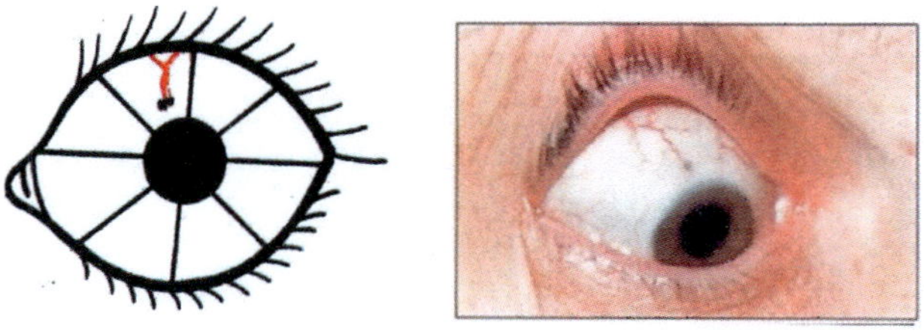

Figure 41 Projecting as a Dewdrop

Color Variances in the Capillary Branches

A. Shades of Red

1. True red: onset of illness and excessive condition
2. Purple-red: more feverish illness
3. Dark red: illness invades into organs, fever progressing
4. Black in with red: Heat developing disorder
5. Yellow in with red: illness getting better

B. Shades of Gray

1. Faded gray: weakness of Qi, lacking of Blood or Cold condition of Qi and Blood stagnation
2. True gray: an old illness

C. Shades of Yellow

1. Yellowish: rate of improvement yet to be determined

By observing the pathological variances of the bulbar conjunctiva capillary branches, practitioners are able to determine the illness Zang or Fu, Yin or Yang, cold or hot, as well as its probable course. The practitioner must rely on what is readily visible when making the decisions. To determine if the illness is in the five Zang, the capillary branches appear transparent in the deep layer, and show as unclear or "foggy". To determine if the illness is in the six Fu, the capillary branches are clearly in the superficial layer. The practitioner continues to observe the evolution of the illness by checking the bulbar capillary branches of the bulbar conjunctiva at each return visit of the patient.

Results of a Double Blind Study in Observation of Ocular Diagnosis

Professor Peng, from 1970 to 1974, researched 10,000 cases using this unique method of recognizing illness by observing the eye for diagnosis. Males and females were equally represented in this double blind research. Ages of those studied were from 25 to 81 years, with the average age between 20 and 50 years. The accuracy of this diagnostic technique between the two groups of observed patients was 90.7%.

CHAPTER SIX

Therapy

In acupuncture theory there are numerous points belonging to the regular channels which are situated around the eye. These points treat various eye conditions and facial problems. Only a few of them are used to treat problems on other parts of the body (i.e., low back pain). The thirteen periocular ocuzones were developed from the Bagua theory and Professor Peng's experience. Their location, effect, indications and puncture methods differ from the standard body of acupuncture knowledge.

The Principle of Selection

- **Selection of the ocuzone along the channel which corresponds with the occurring symptom:**

  First, diagnosis of the patient's symptoms is made and then compared to the channel the symptoms correspond to. Once the illness is determined, select the ocuzone with the same name as the channel. For example, if the patient is coughing, choose the Lung ocuzone; for shoulder pain which involves the Small Intestine channel, select the Small Intestine ocuzone; or, for an occipital headache along the Bladder channel, select the Bladder ocuzone.

- **Selection of ocuzones based on differentiation of the syndrome:**

  Based on the clinical data collected by the four diagnostic methods, determine which Zang-Fu the disease belongs to, then select the corresponding ocuzones for treatment. Let's look at one patient's symptom of "headache" as an example for treatment: upon the evaluation of symptoms, exterior excess syndrome in the Taiyang is determined; the Bladder or Small Intestine ocuzones are then selected. With signs of hyperactivity of Liver Yang, the Liver or Gallbladder zones are selected. With excessive Heat in the Yangming stirring up Wind, Large Intestine and Stomach ocuzones are selected for treatment.

- **Selection of the ocuzone by reference to the exterior-interior relationship:**

  The corresponding ocuzone is selected based upon the subordinate relationship of Zang-Fu or the exterior-interior relationship of the channels. For example: for symptoms appearing in the lung, select the Large Intestine ocuzone.

- **Contralateral acupuncture across the channel:**

  In "Contralateral Acupuncture", *Plain Questions, Yellow Emperor's Canon of Internal medicine*, it says "In contralateral acupuncture, for the left, select the right, for the right, select the left". According to this, when the disease is on the left side of the body, select the right periocular ocuzone.

- **Selection of ocuzones by observing the eye:**

  Carefully observe the pathological and color changes of the ocular conjunctival capillary branches. Find the region with the most prominent changes, then select its corresponding acupuncture ocuzone around the orbit, much as one chooses an Ashi point when doing body acupuncture. It has been this author's experience that this type of selection process can be very effective.

- **Selection of ocuzones according to the location of disease in the Triple-Warmer:**

  Based on the demarcation of the Triple Warmer, the corresponding Upper, Middle, or Lower Warmer ocuzone can be selected. For example, when treating stroke, if the upper and lower extremities show motor dysfunction, selecting either the Upper or Lower Warmer ocuzone for treatment produces a very good result. This mode of selection has been widely chosen by Professor Peng and his students.

The Indications of Periocular Acupuncture and Therapeutic Prescriptions from Dr. Peng's Experience

Periocular acupuncture is used for relief of pain, lessening of swelling, reducing anxiety and calming, eliminating stagnation, regulating the flow of Qi and Blood, clearing and energizing the channels and collaterals, harmonizing and strengthening the functions of the organs and balancing Yin and Yang. As can be seen, periocular acupuncture not only treats the patient's symptoms, but treats the root of the problem as well.

Stroke and Hemiplegia (Zhangfeng and Weizheng)

For newer cases which have already passed through the critical stages of intensive care, puncturing the #5-Upper Warmer ocuzone and the #13-Lower Warmer ocuzone can bring about an instant effect. For those patients with a chronic condition of several months or years, but whose muscles and joints all remain normal, this treatment will still be effective. But in those long standing cases where the muscles have atrophied and the bone has deformed, the movement of the shoulder and the elbow joints are restricted, the feet everted or inverted, or with cerebromalacia or encephalotrophy, the therapeutic effects will mostly be unsatisfactory.

For hemiplegia in the early stage, ask the patient to lie supine and extend the legs. The acupuncturist flexes the patient's knee on the affected side and puts the sole of the foot flat on the bed. If the knee remains upright, the treatment will be effective because the affected side does not show muscle atrophy. Conversely, if the affected leg cannot be kept in a stable and flexed position, the treatment will have little effect.

Professor Peng and his research group have treated 598 cases of stroke patients as of the year 1992. The total effectiveness rate was 94.8%*.

Professor Peng concluded that for stroke resulting from embolism, the sooner the patient received treatment, the better the success. Some patients could even get up from bed after just one treatment, or experienced complete recovery after just 3-5 treatments. The average for the most significant improvement was one month of treatment. If the stroke had been caused by hemorrhage, and the patient had other severe symptoms, Professor Peng usually waited for those symptoms to improve, then chose the periocular needling technique to help the hemiplegia.

*Dr. Tian Weizhu is Professor Peng's best fellowship student. He is one of the directors of the Acupuncture Department and Chief Director of the Ocular Therapy Research Department with the Affiliated Hospital of Liaoning College of TCM. He reported an effective rate of 97.5% in 1993.

Abnormal Blood Pressure

Periocular acupuncture is very good for regulating the blood and is especially effective for lowering high blood pressure. Dr. Tian reported an effectiveness rate of 89% in 1993, selecting #6-Liver ocuzone for straight insertion. An average of 6-10 treatments was required to stabilize the blood pressure to within the normal range. After obtaining a normal level, the continuation of treatments did not cause a further drop in blood pressure. In patients with additional symptoms of dizziness, headache, concentration difficulty, etc., Dr. Tian added the needling of #5-Upper Warmer ocuzone. This technique also works for hypotension. After treatments, the blood pressure was raised to a normal level. In conclusion, periocular acupuncture has bi-directional action on the regulation of abnormal blood pressure bringing both hyper and hypo blood pressure to within the normal range.

Soft Tissue Injury

Periocular acupuncture can be applied as strong stimulation for the movement of stagnant Qi and Blood. It can be used to obtain a high degree of success for the treatment of any acute sprain or strain of the soft tissue.

1. **Acute strain of the low back**: Select #13-Lower Warmer ocuzone bilaterally employing a pricking method or perpendicular insertion or twin needles insertion. Results are usually seen immediately, just after the needles are withdrawn. Some cases required the patient to exercise while the needles are retained.
2. **Stiff neck or neck rigidity**: #5-Upper Warmer ocuzone.

3. **Sprain of the shoulder and arm**: #5-Upper Warmer ocuzone, plus select the ocuzone of the channel involved that has the same name, i.e., pain on the back of the shoulder in the scapular area: select #10-Small Intestine ocuzone.

Bi Syndrome

Based on the Triple Warmer Theory of ocular diagnosis, remarkable results in the treatment of the following different Bi Syndromes have been seen:

1. **Sciatica**: #7-Gallbladder ocuzone.
2. **Shoulder pain**: #5-Upper Warmer and #6-Liver ocuzones.
3. **Numbness in the fingers**: Find out the cause of the numbness based on observation of the pathological variances occurring to the ocular capillary. Next, select the appropriate ocuzones.
4. **Hypochondriac pain and back pain**: #7- Gallbladder ocuzone.

Various Kinds of Pain Relief

1. **Headache**: #5-Upper Warmer ocuzone; for migraine, add #7-Gallbladder ocuzone; for occipital headache, add #4-Bladder ocuzone.
2. **Neck pain**: #5-Upper Warmer and #4-Bladder ocuzone; for tension #6-Liver ocuzone.
3. **Facial pain**: Spastic facial muscle #5-Upper Warmer and #11-Spleen ocuzones; for trigeminal neuralgia: ophthalmic branch #5-Upper Warmer ocuzone and GB1 (Tongziliao); mandibular branch add ST6 (Jiache).
4. **Chest pain**: #5-Upper Warmer and #9-Heart ocuzones.
5. **Back pain**: #5-Upper Warmer and #4-Bladder ocuzones.
6. **Lumbago**: #13-Lower Warmer and #3-Kidney ocuzones.
7. **Pain in leg, knee, heel or foot**: #13-Lower Warmer ocuzone plus the appropriate channel point for the proper sign.

Tremor

1. **Hand tremor:** Based on the diagnosis for a deficiency of Qi in the affected organ, select the same organ ocuzone.
2. **Neck tremor:** #5-Upper Warmer ocuzone.
3. **Tremor caused by writing:** #5-Upper Warmer ocuzone.

Paralysis

1. **Facial palsy:** Both sides of #5-Upper Warmer ocuzones.
2. **Other nerve damage:** Based on the affected location, select using the Triple Warmer theory of ocular diagnosis.

Allergies

1. **Hay fever:** Both sides of #5-Upper Warmer ocuzones.
2. **Asthma:** Both sides of #1-Lung and #5-Upper Warmer ocuzones.
3. **Urticaria and skin rash:** Based on observation of the pathological variances of the ocular capillary, select the affecting ocuzone.

Internal Organ Disorders and Symptoms

1. **Cardiac arrhythmia:** Both sides #9-Heart ocuzones.
2. **Chronic senile bronchitis:** Both sides #1-Lung ocuzones.
3. **Phreospasm:** Both sides #8-Middle Warmer ocuzones.
4. **Stomachache or gastrospasm:** #8-Middle Warmer and #12-Stomach ocuzones.
5. **Cholecystitis:** #7-Gallbladder ocuzone.
6. **Biliary ascariasis:** #6-Liver and #7-Gallbladder ocuzones.
7. **Pancreatitis:** #8-Middle Warmer and #11-Spleen ocuzones.
8. **Vomiting** : #8-Middle Warmer and #12-Stomach ocuzones.
9. **Anorexia:** #12-Stomach ocuzone, add Sifeng (extra point).

10. **Loose Stool or diarrhea**: #2-Large Intestine ocuzone.
11. **Dysentery**: #13-Lower Warmer and #2-Large Intestine ocuzones.
12. **Constipation**: #2-Large Intestine ocuzone; intradermal needling on left abdomen over descending colon.

Urogenital Disorders

1. **Dysmenorrhea**: Both sides #13-Lower Warmer ocuzones.
2. **Menstrual Disorders**: #13-Lower Warmer, #6-Liver, and #3-Kidney ocuzones.
3. **Incontinence or frequent urination**: #13-Lower Warmer, #6-Liver and #3-Kidney ocuzones.
4. **Urolithiasis**: #13-Lower Warmer and #3-Kidney ocuzones.
5. **Prostatitis**: #3-Kidney and #13-Lower Warmer ocuzones for symptom relief.

Mental Problems

1. **Anxiety and panic attack**: Based on the differentiation of the syndrome for five organs; mainly select both sides of #9-Heart and #3-Kidney ocuzones to harmonize the relationship between the heart and the kidney.
2. **Neurasthenia**: #5-Upper Warmer, #3-Kidney and #9-Heart ocuzones.

Diseases of the Sense Organs

By placing needles around the orbit of the eye, the technique for diseases of the sense organs is employed. This technique will produce a strong stimulation affecting the eye and is very beneficial in the treatment of eye problems. The following is Professor Peng's list of eleven kinds of diseases and symptoms that can be treated using this method:

1. **Painful conjunctival congestion**: #6-Liver ocuzone.
2. **Myopia**: #6-Liver ocuzone complemented by Neijingming.

3. **Eyelid ptosis**: #5-Upper Warmer ocuzone.
4. **Sty**: #11 Spleen ocuzone.
5. **Arc-flash conjunctivitis**: #5-Upper Warmer ocuzone.
6. **Rhinitis**: #5-Upper Warmer and #1-Lung ocuzones.
7. **Hoarse voice**: #1-Lung and #5-Upper Warmer ocuzones.
8. **Sore throat**: #1-Lung and #5-Upper Warmer ocuzones.
9. **Glossodynia**: #9-Heart ocuzone.
10. **Toothache**: #5-Upper Warmer ocuzone and TW17 (Yifeng) at the affected site; non-effective for dental cavities.
11. **Deafness, tinnitus**: #6-Liver and #5-Upper Warmer ocuzones.

Experiences of Other Acupuncturists

1. **Acute Cholecyspasm**: #4-Bladder and #5-Upper Warmer ocuzones (experience from Shanghai, China) (See Chapter Eight: Clinical Reports).
2. **Sciatica**: #13-Lower Warmer as the main ocuzone, then locate the channel where the pain is occurring and add the ocuzone point with the same name (i.e., if on the Gallbladder channel, may add #7-Gallbladder ocuzone). This clinical experience came from Guangdong Provincial Hospital of TCM, Guangzhou, China.

Personal Experience - Complicated Symptoms

A patient came in with a long list of complaints (i.e., pain, sleeping disturbance, fatigue, anxiety or depression, digestive or menstrual disorders, etc.). The author chose ocular diagnosis and periocular acupuncture as the first choice to put the patient at ease before developing a more focused treatment plan for the main complaint and root problem. The results were remarkable. The most common ocuzones selected were #3-Kidney, #6-Liver, #9-Heart and #13-Lower Warmer. (See Chapter Eight: Clinical Reports)

CHAPTER SEVEN

Periocular Needling Technique

The gauge of the needle chosen for the periocular needle technique should range from #29 to #34 and be 0.5 cun in length. The patient should be in a supine position. Be sure the patient is calm and comfortable before needling.

Insertion

Follow the procedure for clean needle technique. However, be careful with the use of alcohol because if it comes in contact with the eyeball, it can cause the patient discomfort. The acupuncturist should use the thumb and index fingers of one hand to tighten the eyelid on the selected zone and press the eyeball away to protect it. The other hand is the puncturing hand for inserting the needle. The depth of insertion usually is into the subcutaneous space. Be careful to not touch the eyeball. Be precise and puncture within the ocuzone chosen, making sure you do not cross over the boundary. ***The technique should be steady, accurate, quick and light.***

The Various Puncturing Methods

Tapping Method:

1. With one hand, press the eyelid on the superficial skin area.
2. With the other hand, using a needle, gently tap on the selected ocuzone about 5-7 times, taking precautions against bleeding. The needle should just be touching the skin.

Perpendicular Method:

This insertion should be adjacent to the margin of the ocuzone chosen. The intraorbital needlings are all perpendicular with the needle pointing toward the orbital wall. The insertion should be less than 5 mm. (Figure 42)

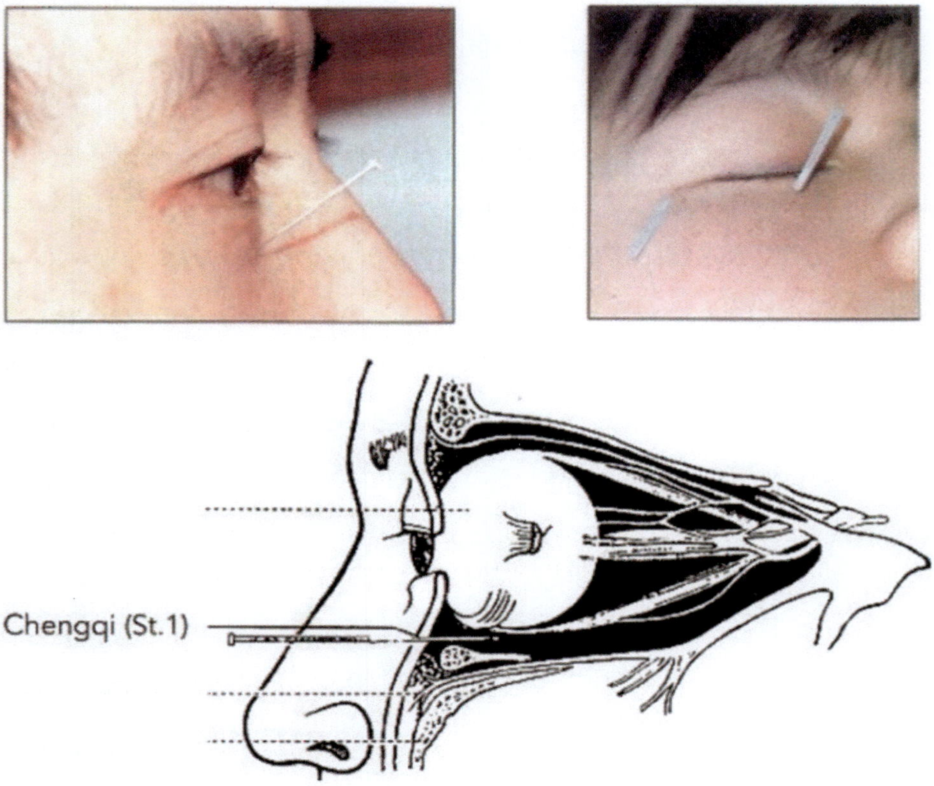

Figure 42 Perpendicular Method

Extraorbital Method:

This is for horizontal insertion. At the selected and well demarcated ocuzone, insert the needle along the skin and in the appropriate direction. The insertion may go as deep, but no deeper, than the subcutaneous tissue. In a two ocuzone region, the insertion should not cross over into the area of the adjacent ocuzone. In the Triple Warmer regions, puncture only one ocuzone in each region. (Figure 43)

Twin Needle Method:

In both perpendicular and horizontal insertions, once a needle is inserted, it is feasible to insert another needle next to it in the same direction. The therapeutic effect may thus be enhanced in this manner. (Figure 43)

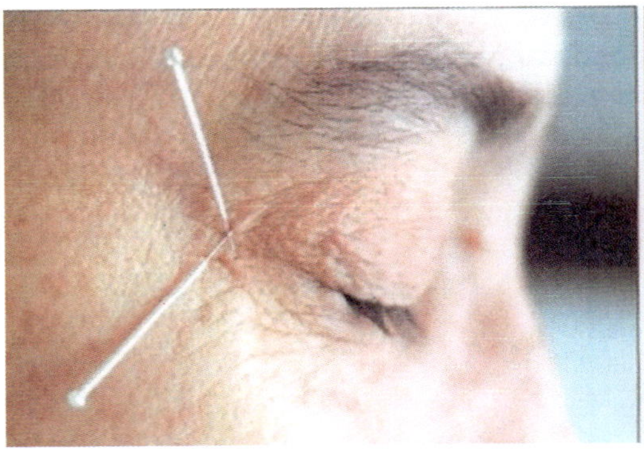

Figure 43 Extraorbital Method

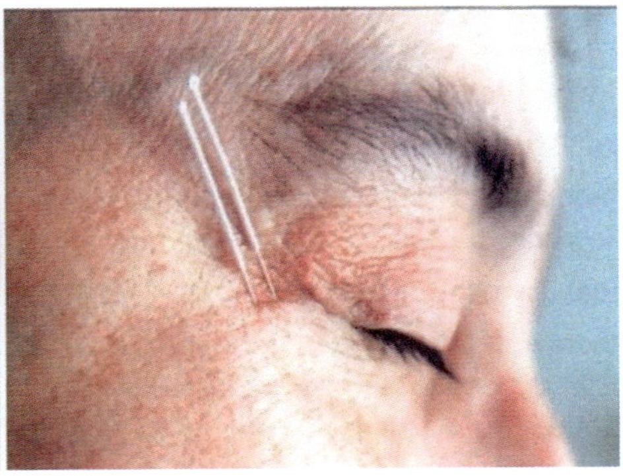

Figure 44 Twin Needle Technique

Inner-outer Combined Method:

At the selected periocular region, insert one needle intraorbitally and one extraorbitally. This combination will usually produce a better effect. (Figure 45)

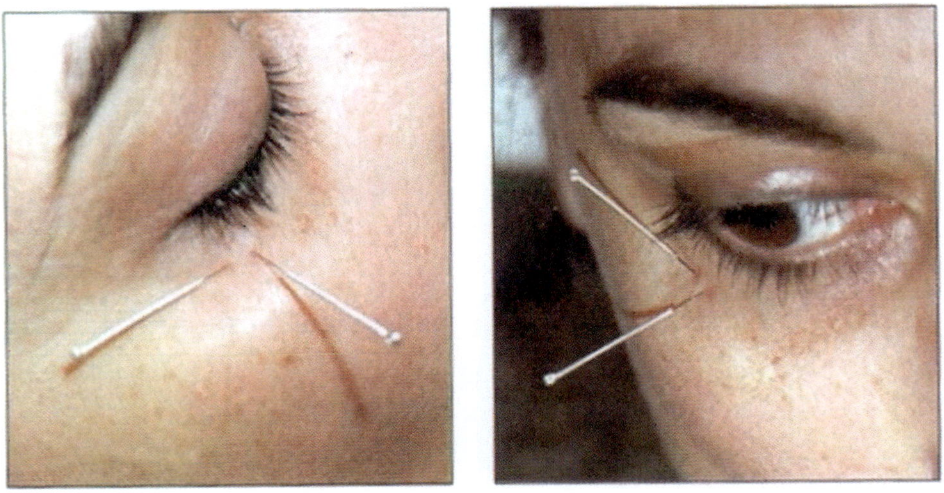

Figure 45 Inner-Outer Combined Method

Ocuzone Acupressure Method:

Press the selected point with a finger until the patient reports a sensation of soreness or numbness. A small glass rod or the handle of a three-edged needle can be used in place of needle insertion with the same effect. In cases of children who are afraid of needling or with individuals who are needle-shy, acupoint pressing may be used effectively.

Embedded Acupuncture:

For those patients with unstable therapeutic results, try implanting a vaccaria seed or an intradermal needle.

Symmetrical Ocuzone Method:

When the disease is on one side of the body and needling on the same side is ineffective, it is possible to needle the same name ocuzone on the eye on opposite side. This method is the based on the same theory as contralateral acupuncture.

Electrical Method:

After the needles have been inserted at the points, attach an electro-acupuncture device and give a continuous impulse to the puncture area. The author used the G6805 machine. For pain relief, put on frequency #5. The intensity is adjusted to the patient's comfort level. This technique is used for a duration of 20 to 30 minutes.

As an adjunct with other therapeutic methods:

Periocular acupuncture can be applied alone or applied in association with other therapy (e.g., body acupuncture, scalp acupuncture, plum-blossom needling, auricular acupuncture, intradermal needling, massage, Qigong, medication and various physical therapies).

Needle Manipulation

Periocular acupuncture does not need manipulation such as lifting and thrusting or twisting and twirling. If the Qi does not arrive, lift the needle halfway up and insert at another angle; or scratch the needle handle lightly to enhance the effect.

Needle Retention

Professor Peng suggested that the needle be retained and undisturbed after the Qi has arrived for 5 to 15 minutes. The author usually retains the needles a bit longer because patients are in a lying down, relaxed position. It is different than in China where patients are sitting upright in a busy treatment room.

Withdrawal of Needle

The technique should be slow and light. At first swing the needle handle lightly, then gradually lift the needle up halfway. Wait for a moment, then pull the needle out and immediately press on the site with a small sterilized cotton ball for 2 to 3 minutes.

Contraindications

Periocular acupuncture technique is not contraindicated unless the patient is critical or irritable. For patients with thickened or congested eyelids, the technique should not be applied.

Tips on the Method

Clinically, in selecting the thirteen ocuzones the application of the following three methods are of great importance for the practitioner who is not familiar with this technique.

1. With a thin glass rod or the handle of a three edged needle, apply even and light pressure around the orbital regions. The response of the localities may be soreness, numbness, distention, heaviness or heat, cold sensation, slight pain or just discomfort.

   Once having found a responsive location, increase the pressure slightly to form a small dimple to mark the site for acupuncture. Some patients may have no responding sensations and in this case, just barely insert the needle at the selected ocuzone.

2. Select the point with an acupoint detector.

3. Once the point to be needled is determined, locate the ocuzone accurately by using the pupil as the reference center while having the patient look straight forward. Apply perpendicular or horizontal needle insertion at the ocuzone.

Ten Precautionary Measures

The unique application and therapeutic effect of periocular acupuncture developed by Professor Peng Jingshan has been widely recognized. It is undeniable that this method is gaining recognition the world over and is being accepted by both acupuncturists and their patients. However, in promoting this method, it may cause fear and doubt in the patient if one overlooks the fact that this therapy may easily cause bleeding after application. If bruising and swelling around the eyes occur after treatment, this may cause distress to the patient and a sense of guilt and regret for the acupuncturist. So, taking precautionary measures regarding the application of this method is very important.

1. If the patient has fear and doubt about this method, resists the idea or has no confidence in the acupuncturist, it is best to give more thought before employing this technique. Avoid making a quick decision that may not be appropriate.

2. Patients who are emotionally unstable, especially those who have been crying prior to treatment, should refrain from having immediate treatment by this method.

3. Those patients with clotting mechanism disorders, such as hemophilia, diabetes, those taking anticoagulants on a long term basis, and elderly people who take aspirin daily, should receive this treatment with extra caution and care.
4. Acupuncturists who are not familiar with the anatomy of the eye, especially regarding innervation and the path of blood vessels within the orbit and the eyelids, should study the anatomy afresh before applying this method.
5. Those who are new to the profession or who are not familiar with this method should first practice on a model until they are comfortable with the technique and before they undertake clinical practice.
6. When the treatment room is not adequately lit or the acupuncturist has sight problems, the conditions need to be remedied to a suitable level before applying periocular acupuncture.
7. If the patient is not lying comfortably or if the patient cannot remain at rest for at least 15 minutes while undergoing acupuncture, this method should not be applied. For example, when a patient has a serious cough.
8. When the needle is inserted and retained, pressure should not be applied to the soft tissues surrounding the eye area or to the eye muscles. While the needle is retained, the patient should refrain from chatting, coughing, sneezing or making sudden movements, etc. As for patients suffering partial paralysis after a stroke, or those with a frozen shoulder, the affected limb should be moved to complement the therapy after insertion of the needles. However, under no circumstances should pressure be added to the eye region.
9. Do not immediately send the patient off after withdrawing the needles. Upon withdrawal, the acupuncturist should lightly press a small sterile cotton ball to the needled area for 2 to 3 minutes. This is also the time to check for bleeding, and explain to the patient about appropriate precautionary measures.
10. The patient should avoid strenuous exercise or heavy manual labor right both after the treatment and the following day. The patient should also be warned not to use the hands, fingers, tissues or towels

to rub his/her eye because rubbing the eye after acupuncture may lead to bleeding.

Conclusion: If these ten precautionary measures are closely observed, most complications can be prevented. The therapeutic effect of periocular acupuncture will be enhanced and its clinical relevancy will be promoted, aided by acupuncturists working to diminish the occurrence of complications.

CHAPTER EIGHT

Clinical Reports

Reviewing academic journals for published clinical studies in ocular acupuncture, the author was unable to find much information in this field. She found those studies dealt mostly with treatment for pain, (i.e., shoulder pain, low back pain, sciatica, cholecystitis and asthma). For purposes of this chapter, Professor Peng's typical cases and other reports from his *Ocular Acupuncture* book have been selected for the reader's review.

Professor Peng's Report of 13 Typical Cases

1. **Lung ocuzone for treatment of skin rash in a 19 year old female:** TCM determined the problem to be Heat in the lungs. The diagnosis was erysipelas. The patient had a fever of 39°C with no response to antibiotics. Her WBC count was 15,300. The differential of WBC showed the neutrophil cell count was 85% before treatment. After only one periocular treatment, her WBC dropped to 10,000 with a neutrophil cell count of 61%. The fever was also gone. Only 3 treatments were needed to cure the problem.
2. **Large Intestine ocuzone for chronic diarrhea in a 42 year old female:** The chronic diarrhea was due to deficiency and cold in the abdomen after a stomach operation and duodenectomy. The condition had lasted for two years and the patient was very thin and weak. After one periocular acupuncture treatment, the abdominal pain and diarrhea stopped. The patient had a series of 13 treatments resulting in recovery of her basic health.
3. **Kidney ocuzone treating acute low back strain in a 47 year old male:** The patient's back was very rigid with little range of motion. After the needles were inserted using periocular acupuncture, there was

immediate relief from pain and a return to a full range of motion in his waist and back. In a follow up with the patient a few days later, he reported no recurrence of the problem.

4. **Bladder ocuzone for haematuria in a 45 year old male:** The patient had been diagnosed with haematuria which had lasted for several years. He had seen and been treated by many doctors, but with no results. After five periocular acupuncture treatments, the blood in his urine was almost gone. The patient had three more treatments. A lab report one month later showed that his urinalysis was once again normal.

5. **Upper Warmer ocuzone for hemiplegia in a 58 year old male:** A stroke six months earlier had left the patient unable to raise his left arm. After one periocular acupuncture treatment, he was able to move his arm up one foot. After only two treatments, the paralyzed arm could be raised up to head level. Even his primary care physicians were surprised by this fast response.

6. **Liver ocuzone for accumulated Heat in the liver causing lumbago in a 67 year old female:** The patient had chronic lung and heart disease. She was treated at her home because of severe pain and circulatory problems. She could only be treated in a kneeling position on a pillow in bed. After five minutes of treatment using periocular acupuncture, the patient was able to sit up freely. The pain was gone, and she started talking and laughing. She then walked outside with Professor Peng to her gate to thank him for coming to her home to give the treatment. This case had been followed for over six years, and no such pain returned.

7. **Gallbladder ocuzone for pain caused from cholecysitis in a 58 year old male:** The patient had been suffering on and off for one year from pain caused by cholecysitis. During his first treatment he experienced an acute attack. Five minutes after the needles were inserted using periocular acupuncture, the pain was gone. All symptoms disappeared at the end of six treatments.

8. **Middle Warmer ocuzone for phrenospasm in a 74 year old male:** The patient had severe spasming in his diaphragm for many days. Professor

Peng's treatment brought the spasming under control after only three treatments. The patient had a total of six treatments and recovered fully.

9. **Heart ocuzone for continuous violent palpitations caused by coronary heart disease in a 47 year old male:** After needle insertion, the patient's chest felt more comfortable. The symptoms were gone after 12 periocular acupuncture treatments.

10. **Small Intestine ocuzone for upper abdominal pain due to postoperative rupture of the duodenum in a 28 year old male**: The pain was relieved after two periocular acupuncture treatments. The patient fully recovered after six treatments, and reported having more strength than before the surgery.

11. **Spleen ocuzone for phrenospasm due to Spleen Qi deficiency in a 38 year old male**: The patient had the problem for 20 years. The spasm occurred monthly usually lasting seven to eight days. The patient had been treated by numerous methods, all of which failed. When the patient came to see Professor Peng during an attack, the spasm stopped immediately after the insertion of needles.

12. **Stomach ocuzone for severe stomach pain due to Cold accumulation and Qi stagnation in a 35 year old male**: The patient was in great pain when he presented for treatment. After needle insertion, his stomach pain was gone. Follow ups showed no reoccurrence of pain.

13. **Lower Warmer ocuzone for a cerebrovascular accident in a 43 year old female:** The patient had received periocular acupuncture treatment from Professor Peng the day after her stroke. Initially the patient's right side was totally paralyzed. After needle insertion, the right arm and leg started to move. Professor Peng then asked her to get up from her bed. With the needles still retained and someone's help, the patient started walking firmly while carrying her intravenous bottle. There were more than ten people in the hospital room who witnessed the patient walking again just after the periocular needles were inserted in the Lower Warmer zones. The patient was discharged from the hospital the next day and returned for four more treatments. The patient was able to return to work after two months and felt as

healthy as she was before the stroke. Professor Peng stressed that this was but one of a number of successful cases. Many stroke patients who were treated in the early stages obtained the same beneficial results.

Periocular Acupuncture for Cholecyspasm

250 cases of acute pain from gallbladder spasm were treated with periocular needle technique by Dr. Wang Zhihua and others at the Shanghai First People's Hospital. This author and his practicing group are M.D.'s who basically practice Western medicine. There were 122 cases of gallbladder spasm caused by cholelithiasism that were diagnosed by ultrasound. Analysis was based on these 122 cases.

There were 99 female and 23 male patients with ages ranging from 30 to 82 years old. 99 out of 122 patients had gallstones located inside the gallbladder. In 7 cases, the gallstones were located in the liver. In 6 cases, the gallstones were lodged in the gallbladder duct.

All patients presented as emergency cases. 62.4% obtained immediate pain relief within five minutes after needle insertion. 35.5% felt greatly improved and 2% felt no change after treatment. After observing the patients for two days, 16.8% still felt the same level of pain, 19% felt discomfort in the gallbladder region, and for 63.6%, the pain was completely gone with no recurrent symptoms. After only one treatment and a one month follow-up, 30 cases had no symptoms. Selections were regions IV and V using horizontal insertion at 2 mm outside the orbit edge. #30 gauge and 0.5 inch needles were used.

Manipulation was not needed. The direction of the needle followed clockwise on the left eye and counterclockwise on the right eye. The needles were retained for 5 minutes.

30 cases in the control group were treated by medication (Atropine, Dilantin IV, 654-2, etc). The shortest time until relief in this group was 9 minutes, and the longest time was 35 minutes. The average time was 20 minutes. This was a great difference when compared to the periocular needled group.

The author suggested that the periocular needling technique is a simple and fast treatment for relieving cholecyspasm pain. After the pain is relieved, antibiotics should still be used to control any infection in the gallbladder.

Clinical Research on Ocular Diagnosis and Periocular Acupuncture Treatments

This article was written by Dr. Zhu Jiang, *et.al.* of Beijing College of TCM, China. Professor Peng was their supervisor. The following is a summary of their research:

Three Methods of Diagnosis Used:

Method 1 - Ocuzone's pathological changes on the conjunctiva.

Method 2 - Using an electrical device (TJ-1 Taiji Brand developed in Chinese Science College) to check for sensitive points around the orbit.

Method 3 - Using the TJ-1 to check for low electrical resistance points on the ears.

The three methods produced the following results in diagnostic accuracy:

Method 1: 75% accurate in 36 out of 48 cases.

Method 2: 82% accurate in 24 out of 29 cases.

Method 3: 64% accurate in 16 out of 25 cases.

- **Relationship of the three methods of diagnosis with pain:** Method 1: 76% effective in 16 out of 21 cases. Method 2: 75% effective in 9 out of 12 cases. Method 3: 73% effective in 8 out of 11 cases.
- **Relationship of the three methods of diagnosis in stroke patients**: Method 1: 75% effective in 6 out of 8 cases. Method 2: 67% effective in 2 out of 3 cases. Method 3: 62% effective in 5 out of 8 cases

- **Relationship of the three methods of diagnosis on the same patients:** No difference shown.

Periocular Acupuncture Treatment for Pain Relief:

- Immediate response was 53% in 10 out 19 cases.
- After patients had completed a series of treatments the result was 95% effectiveness resulting in 18 out of 19 cases.Periocular Acupuncture Treatment for Hemiplegia Patients:
- Immediate response was 86% in 6 out of 7 cases.
- There was a result of 100% effectiveness, or 7 out of 7, after patients had completed the series of treatment.

Periocular Acupuncture Treatment for Patients with High Blood Pressure:

- Immediate response was 50% of 2 out of 4 cases.
- There was a result of 75% effectiveness or 3 out of 4 cases after patients had completed the series of treatment.

The author concluded that those patients who finished the series of treatments obtained the most successful results.

Ocular Diagnosis and Periocular Acupuncture for Complicated Symptoms

Dr. Hoy Ping Yee Chan wanted to obtain better results towards full recovery for patients suffering complicated symptoms resulting from physical or emotional trauma. Periocular acupuncture is designed for treatment of such symptoms. During early visits, patients often presented with a long list of complaints. Before targeting a focused treatment for their main complaints, patients should be calm and put at ease, the acupuncturist treating the body as a whole during the first few visits. If this therapeutic approach is used before focusing on the chief complaint and treating the root problem, the results can be remarkable.

Method: The following explains how Professor Peng Jingshan's Ocular Diagnosis and his unique needling technique were used to treat complicated conditions.

First, the patient's health condition was determined by observing the bulbar conjunctiva of the eyes. All patients were noted as having abnormal pathologic changes on the capillary branches which appeared as an enlargement of the capillaries or capillary twisting; some of them showed thick stems or having many small bifurcating branches. A blurred area appeared in the Liver zone on the patients suffering from emotional stress or depression. The color of the capillaries had changed to bright red, indicating the conditions were newly generated and of an excess nature.

Second, needles of #32 gauge, length 0.5 inch, were applied bilaterally on the abnormal zones. Two to four pairs of ocuzones were selected from those regions. The most common zones were #3-Kidney, #4-Bladder, #6-Liver, #9-Heart and #13-Lower Warmer. The insertion technique had to be steady, accurate, quick and light. The needles were retained for 20 to 30 minutes. Manipulation to the needles was not needed after the Qi arrived. During the treatment most patients felt comfortable and relaxed while the needles were retained. The withdrawal of the needles was gentle, followed by light pressure applied on the zones against the orbit using small sterile cotton balls. No pressure was applied to the eyeballs. Important precautionary measures were used due to the probability of bleeding after application. (Figure 46)

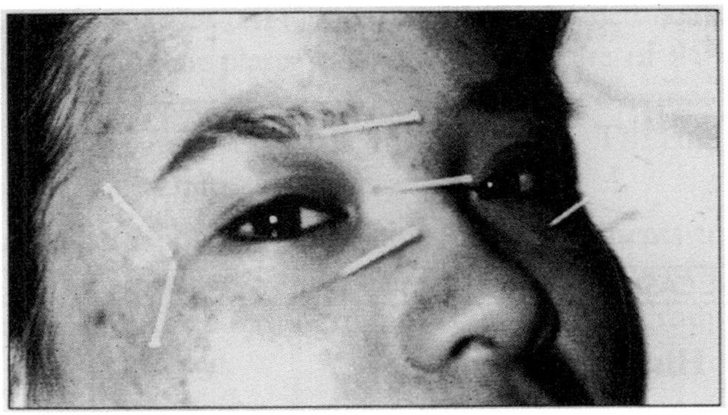

Figure 46 Patient with Complicated Symptoms Receiving Periocular Acupuncture Treatment

Results: Thirty-three cases were diagnosed and treated with this method between the period of October 1992 to April 1996. The control group, patients with similar chief complaints but without complicated symptoms, were randomly selected from the computer's data reports during the time period. *97% of the 33 patients obtained relief of complicated symptoms. They were calmer, slept better, and felt overall improvement within one to three visits. There was *1 individual who discontinued treatment after 5 intermittent visits. In the control group, **67% of 33 patients showed improvement within the first three visits. There were **11 cases who had discontinued treatment. The results marked with * and ** are discussed in the Conclusion section on the next page.

Of the thirty-two cases receiving periocular acupuncture, those who completed the treatment plans had an effectiveness rate of 94%. This percentage refers to the relief of the complicated symptoms and the chief complaints and some of the root problems. The comparative control group effectiveness rate was 91%.

The follow up reports (done three months later) of patients treated by periocular acupuncture showed a long term effectiveness of 91%. The effectiveness rate for the control group was 90%. Each group had ten evaluation sheets returned.

The Tables 2 and 3 show the other analytical data.

Conclusion: The eyes have a very close relationship to the body. There are eight regular meridians which have direct contact with the eyes and all twelve regular meridians are connected through the internal-external relationship. Six out of eight extra channels, the muscular regions, and five organs all influence the eyes. All these result in the flow of Qi to the eyes. Needle stimulation to the periocular zones moves and invigorates the Qi, promotes blood circulation, balances Zang-Fu function, and thus benefits the body's recovery from illness.

Professor Peng Jingshan used periocular acupuncture to treat numerous health disorders, but did not mention using this technique for treating complicated symptom presentations in his practice. Periocular acupuncture was chosen for my practice here in the United States to treat those patients with more complicated symptoms. My patients and I are very satisfied with the results.

		Treatment Group	Control Group
SEX	Male	10	13
	Female	23	20
AGE	Under 20	2	1
	21 - 30	1	6
	31 - 40	12	7
	41 - 50	11	7
	51 -60	2	5
	Above 61	5	7
CHIEF COMPLAINT	Back Pain	7	7
	Knee Pain	3	3
	Leg Pain	3	3
	Neck Pain	1	1
	Hand Pain	1	1
	Headache	1	1
	Sciatica	1	1
	Fatigue	7	7
	Digestion Problem	4	4
	Sleeping Problem	2	2
	Anxiety	1	1
	High Blood Pressure	1	1
	Eye Problem	1	1
TOTAL CASES		33	33

Table 2: General Data

PHYSICAL	Car Accident	8
	Surgery	7
	Soft Tissue Strain	3
EMOTIONAL	Stress	12
	Worry	3
	Depression	4
	Fear	1
TOTAL CASES	33: 5 Cases with both trauma	38

Table 3: History of Trauma

The remarkable difference in results between the treatment group and the control group was seen most significantly during the first three treatments. *97% of the periocular acupuncture patients felt better and noticed considerable benefit from the treatments. Hence, they stayed and finished the treatment plan. In the control group, there were **33% of 33 patients who discontinued treatment within the first three visits. As a result, they lost the chance to obtain a full recovery. Although the effectiveness rates for the patients in both groups showed no significant difference, the results indicate that if the patients had stayed for a full treatment series, they would have received satisfactory results. The periocular treatment patient group had many complicated symptoms involving both physical and emotional trauma. These patients were more difficult to treat, yet successful results were achieved.

Clinical Reports from Dr. Hoy Ping Yee Chan

In my clinical practice in Seattle, hundreds of patients have received the benefits of this unique acupuncture technique, especially patients presenting with complicated symptoms. The following is a compilation of feelings and reactions they have shared regarding periocular needling treatment and the beneficial results obtained.

Case 1:

C.N. is a 44 years old female teacher. Her first visit was March 23,1994. She was referred to this clinic by her family physician. She was diagnosed with hyperthyroidism and had an operation for a partial thyroidectomy. A few months after surgery, the patient was still experiencing many of the same symptoms (i.e., anxiety, nausea, diarrhea, an overactive appetite with continued weight loss, insomnia and fatigue). Her blood tests were slightly higher than the normal range T4: 12.8. Her tongue was red at the tip and the edges had a yellow coat. Her pulse was weak in the kidney position and the other pulses were tight. In traditional Chinese medicine the diagnosis was deficiency of Heart Yin, Yangming Syndrome and phlegm stagnation. After a series of nine treatments, all her symptoms were under control, and her blood tests were back to a normal level. The patient returned for a series of six and ten treatments in 1995 and 1996 when she experienced tension, irritation and disturbed sleep. Her other symptoms have not recurred since 1994, and her blood test results have stayed within normal range. Both she and her doctor are pleased with her results from periocular acupuncture. These treatments helped her avoid further radical medical treatments such as radiation. Here is how she describes her periocular needling treatment:

"A minute or two after the needles are in, I begin to slowly feel more and more relaxed until I am extremely relaxed. I normally feel quite tense most of the time. I also usually have trouble getting to sleep at night and wake up easily. But after the treatment, I am able to sleep much more easily. I also feel calmer during the day and have better energy."--C.N.

Case 2:

School teacher L.W.A. is a 45 year old female. She was under a lot of emotional stress from her family and work. Her first visit, on June 25, 1987, was for neck and shoulder pain. She returned on and off for treatments using body acupuncture and had a great deal of symptom relief. Recently, after a divorce trauma, her symptoms became more complicated. She had a tight liver pulse, a red tongue without coating, a flaring-up Liver Fire and Yin deficiency. Periocular acupuncture was chosen for treatment. She feels this technique is different from the body acupuncture and had this to say:

"Dr. Chan gently and delicately inserted the fine needles at points around my eyes. There was a slight tingling sensation upon insertion of the needles, but there was no pain. After the eye needles were in place, I felt tension releasing from my head and neck muscles, and energy flowing down both arms through my finger tips. I became relaxed and felt "lighter". As I sat up after the treatment, I felt rested as if from a long sleep. That evening, I continued to feel "renewed" and slept soundly. The next day, my sinuses were clear, my eyes did not ache, and I continued to have relief from the neck and shoulder tension." --L.W.A.

Case 3:

C.J.B. is a General Manager of a company. She is 45 years old and has felt fatigue for three years. She was diagnosed and treated for hypothyroidism by her family physician. Her other symptoms included indigestion, bloating with gas, loose bowel movements, sleeping disturbance, menopause, low back pain and being overweight. She came to our center for treatment on July 12, 1996. After receiving six ocular acupuncture treatments, she wrote:

"After each acupuncture treatment I've had with Dr. Chan, I have felt more energetic and have clearer vision. She used a technique of needles around the eyes which seems to be working for me. Dr. Chan has the understanding and the sensitivity to do the best she can for her patients. I would recommend her and this kind of treatment to anyone."--C.J.B.

Case 4:

B.F., a 36 year old female who works as a newspaper publisher, was referred to our clinic by her family physician to be treated for arthritis, neck and back pain. She came for her first visit on July 24, 1996. Her other symptoms included stress, fatigue, digestive and hormonal problems, as well as being overweight all her life. Her sedentary work situation caused added stress to her lower back. Fortunately, she had a rapid response to the periocular acupuncture treatments and said the following:

"During the course of four appointments with Dr. Chan, I received acupuncture three times around my eyes and once locally on my back, hip and leg. Dr. Chan inserted the needles around my eyes in several locations. Her "low-key" style is reassuring and inspires trust. Her touch is gentle and imparts a clear sense of genuine concern.

At the initiation of the treatment, I felt a rush of energy which ran through my body, down my arms and legs. Once the needles were in place, I rested and felt very relaxed. After the fourth treatment, I felt more energetic and also the pain in my back had been lessened, which allows me to sleep more comfortably. I attribute this to the care I've received from Dr. Chan, and I look forward to continued improved health under her care."-B.F.

As a unique acupuncture technique, our patients' testimonies prove it to be a very comfortable, calming and an effective therapeutic treatment.

CHAPTER NINE

Prevention: Periocular Self Care

The author would like to take this opportunity to share her experience on how to use periocular self care for disease prevention purposes. Although many people think they are healthy and feel no need for acupuncture treatment, an imbalance in the energy may exist, and underlying disorders may be present. It is important to follow this rule: treat symptoms as early as possible and prevent disease before it happens. It is very important for healthcare practitioners to educate patients on how to do so. The following are some effective periocular self care techniques.

Periocular Acupressure by Finger

The thumb or index fingertip, with a well trimmed nail, should be placed just below the medial upper eyebrow. Gently put pressure on the base of the upper edge of the palpebrae and slowly, evenly, move the finger tip from medial to lateral under the eyebrow, to the lower palpebrae. Pressure should be on the edge of the orbital bone, not on the eyeball. If any soreness or tenderness is discovered, these are the points upon which acupressure is applied, for about one minute. Repeat the acupressure daily until the soreness or tenderness disappears.

A Smooth Round Tip Probe

A glass probe (Figure 48) or any other kind of material bar as long as the tip is smooth with a round shape, can be used in place of the finger to press on the soreness or tender ocuzones.

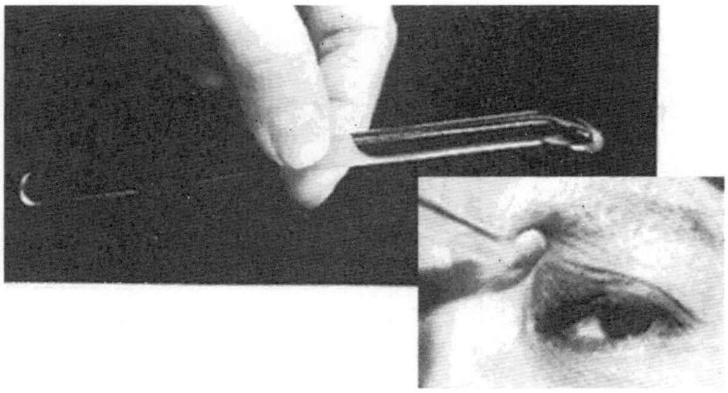

Figure 48 Glass Probe

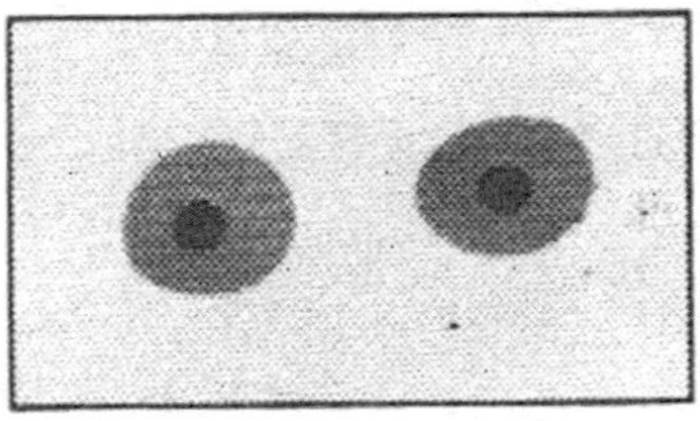

Figure 49 Ferrite Magnets

A Ferrite Magnet

A therapeutic magnetic device such as a ferrite magnet can be placed on an area of the skin. The author prefers a small size (800 gauge ferrite; 0.12" diameter X 0.05" thick) hand magnet such as in Figure 49, which is made in Korea. It is very easy to use. The south pole of the magnet is positioned on the surface of the skin, and its magnetic waves stimulate the Qi and Blood to relieve the blockage. It may be placed on the sore or tender ocuzone before retiring for the night, and removed upon rising. It is fine to apply more than one magnet. The magnets are reusable.

A Magnetic Blunt-tip Needle

A magnetic blunt tip needle is designed especially for self care. It applies pressure to the acupoint while at the same time sends an invisible magnetic force to the body, therefore exerting a double effect. It comes in different styles. There are two kinds shown in Figure 50 - one looks like a pen, the other is on a key chain.

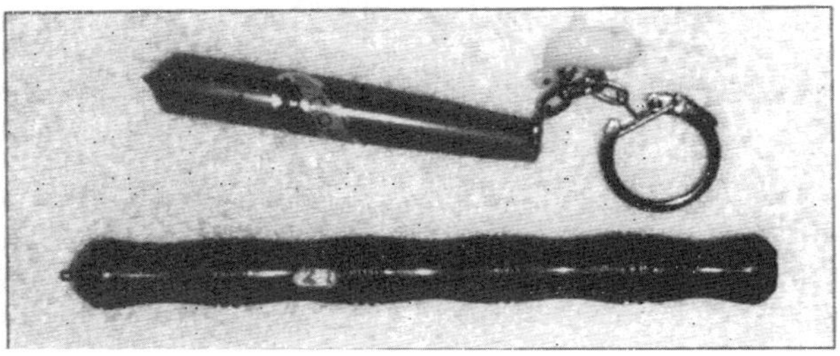

Figure 50 Magnetic Blunt-Tip Needles

References

1. 眼針療法: 彭靜山著
2. 中醫眼科學: 廣州中醫學院主編
3. 中醫眼科學: 廖品正主編
4. 中國醫學百科全書之一一; 中醫眼科學: 陸南山
5. 現代眼科手冊: 楊鈞主編
6. 眼科科學: 毛文書主編
7. 眼科臨床實踐: 天津市眼科醫院主編
8. 實用針灸療法大全: 府強主編編
9. 漢英常用中醫詞彙: 北京醫學院謝竹藩主編編
10. 簡明中醫辭典: << 中醫辭典>> 編輯委員會編
11. 彭靜山教授治學經驗及對醫學的貢獻: 遼寧中醫學院田維柱
12. Peng, Jingshan, Lecture: "Ocular Acupuncture Therapy (1)", *International Journal of Clinical Acupuncture*, Vol.4, No.1, 1993
13. Peng, Jingshan, Lecture: "Ocular Acupuncture Therapy (2)", *International Journal of Clinical Acupuncture*, Vol. 4, No. 2, 1993
14. Dale, Ralph Alan, Ed.D., Ph.D., C.A., Dipl. Ac., *The Principles and Clinical Applications of the Triple Warmer and the Five Phases in Eye Orbit Micro-Acupuncture*
15. O'Connor, John & Bensky, Dan, Translated and Edited, *Acupuncture, A Comprehensive Text*, Shanghai College of Traditional Medicine
16. Cheng, Xiannong, Chief Editor, *Chinese Acupuncture and Moxibustion*, Foreign Languages Press, Beijing

17. The Academy of Traditional Chinese Medicine, *An Outline of Chinese Acupuncture*

18. Clemente, Carmine D., *Anatomy, A Regional Atlas of the Human Body*, 2nd Edition Urban Schwarzenberg

19. Gray, Henry, F.R.S., *Anatomy, Descriptive and Surgical*

20. Amadon, Alfred Mason, M.D., *The Fold-Out Atlas of the Human Body*

About the Author

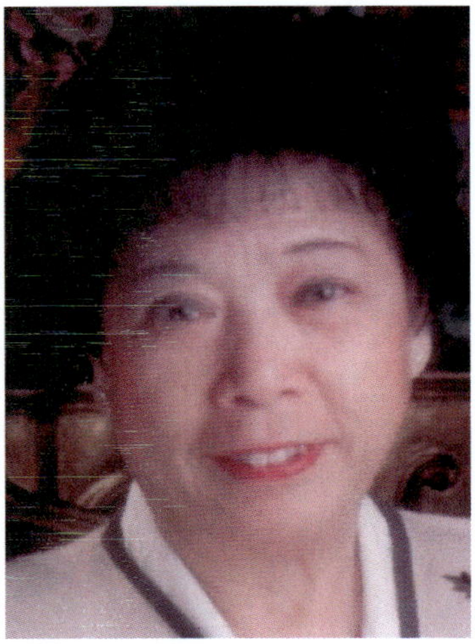

Hoy Ping Yee Chan 陳余海平中醫針灸師, OMD, L.Ac. (Retired NCCAOM), was one of the first independent acupuncture practitioners in Washington State when the bill legalizing acupuncture was passed in 1985. She holds a doctoral degree in Oriental Medicine from SAMRA University in Los Angeles, U.S.A. Before immigrating to America, she practiced Western medicine in China for 18 years after graduation from Beijing (Peking) Medical University.

Within the last thirty years, Dr. Chan has shared her theories, medical knowledge, clinical experience and health care recommendations in acupuncture schools, continuing education seminars, televisions, newspaper interviews, public communities, as well as made presentations at acupuncture conferences worldwide.

In 1996, Dr. Chan compiled the first edition of *Window of Health---Ocular Diagnosis and Periocular Acupuncture,* published by Northwest Institute of Acupuncture and Oriental Medicine. She was one of the first few acupuncturists in U.S. to learn this unique advanced micro-acupuncture technique and tried her best to spread it around the nation.

In 2006, the first issue of *Acupuncture for Stroke Rehabilitation* was published by Blue Poppy Press. Dr. Chan was the chief compiler on the selections of three decades of information from numerous acupuncture and Chinese medical magazines. This is the first book about acupuncture for stroke written in English and includes understanding stroke in Chinese medicine, clinical acupuncture treatments for stroke rehabilitation, various special acupuncture techniques to treat specific post-stroke symptoms, Western medical researchers on acupuncture treatments and stroke prevention information.

In 2007, a special issue of the book *Acupuncture in the Whole World* was published by World Journal of Acupuncture-Moxibustion. In it, Hoy Ping Yee Chan was selected in the outstanding persons list - a great honor to her.

In 2014 Dr. Chan, with her colleague Carole Conlon, published a new book *Chinese Medicine for Aging Eyes*. In this book, she shares her experience in acupuncture and herbal treatments with younger practitioners for the benefit of their eye patients, providing them with material about common eye diseases of seniors beyond what they were taught in school.

Although Dr. Chan has retired from clinical practice, she hopes this resharing of *Window of Health,* along with Dr. Chen's expanded information on the periocular acupuncture technique, will continue to bring this unique technique to younger practitioners and benefit their patients.

Addendum

Chinese Periocular Acupuncture (CPA) and Chinese Periocular Tuina (CPT)

by Y.M. Chen, Ph.D. (OM), L.Ac.

Based Evidence of Chinese Medicine for Eyes

1. Differentiation of Eye Types, Diagnoses (DXs) and Treatments (TXs)
2. Periocular Acupuncture DXs and TXs for Post Traumatic Injury Syndrome (PTIS)
3. Chinese Periocular Tuina (CPT)
4. Preventive Eye Care

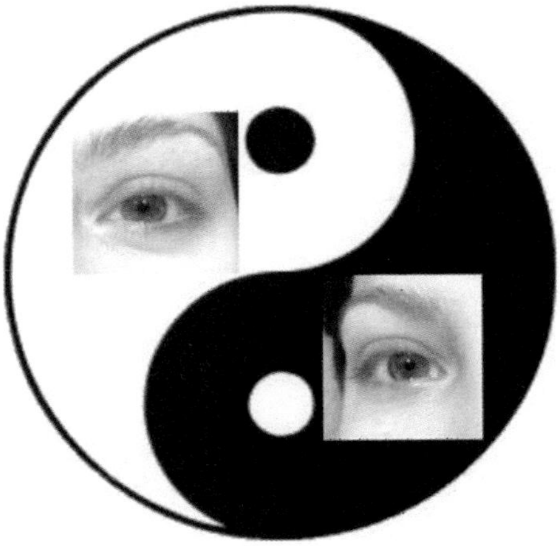

Addendum Figure 1 The Yin/Yang Symbol of Chinese Periocular Acupuncture

Left eye is Yang 左陽, Right eye is Yin 右陰
Created by Y.M. Chen, Ph.D (OM), L.Ac.

What Chinese Medicine Says about Our Eyes

- **The eye is the Window of Health,** 眼睛是健康的窗口
- **The eye is the Window of the Heart and Soul,** 眼睛是心靈之窗
- **The eye functions as the Window of Body Clock,** 眼睛是人體生物鐘
- **The eyes connect to all meridians,** 眼睛連接所有經脈
- **The eye is a part of the central nervous system (Brain and Spinal cord),** 眼睛是中樞神經系統的一部分(大腦和脊髓)
- **The eye is closely linked to and communicating with the liver,** 眼睛與肝藏有密切的聯繫和溝通
- **The eye indicates the balance between the liver (Wood) and the heart (Fire),** 眼睛顯示肝藏和心藏之間的平衡
- **The eye is the thermostat of the blood,** 眼睛是血液的恆溫器
- **The eye is the director of every aspect of life,** 眼睛是生活的各個方面的主管
- **The eye is closely related to our inner consciousness,** 眼睛與我們的內心意識有密切關糸
- **The eyes represent the oracles of a variety of systemic conditions,** 眼睛可反映体內各系统狀態的甲骨文

Five Types of Eyes

1. Angry eyes - Liver, 肝眼
2. Unhappy eyes - Heart, 心眼
3. Worry eyes - Spleen, 脾眼
4. Grief eyes - Lungs, 肺眼
5. Fear eyes - Kidney, 腎眼

Secondary Eye Dysfunctions

1. Strained eye, 緊張的眼
2. Eye allergies - Itchy, red, swollen and tearing, 過敏性眼病
3. Pink eye, 紅眼病
4. Black eye, 黑眼圈

5. Injured eye, 受傷的眼睛

Key Words and Abbreviations

1. CPA – Chinese Periocular Acupuncture - 中醫眼周針療法
2. CPT - Chinese Periocular Tuina - 中醫眼周推拿療法
3. OID - Ocular Inspection and Diagnosis - 眼診斷
4. Ocular Treatment – OT - 眼治療
5. OM – Ocular Melanoma - 眼黑色素癌症腫瘤
6. Liver/Gallbladder ocuzones – LV/GB - 肝膽區
7. Heart/Small Intestine ocuzones – HT/SI - 心小腸區
8. Spleen/Stomach ocuzones – SP/ST - 脾胃區
9. Lung/Large Intestine ocuzones – LU/LI - 肺大腸區
10. Kidney/Bladder ocuzones – KI/BL - 腎膀胱區
11. Upper Warmer – UW - 上焦區
12. Middle Warmer – MW - 中焦區
13. Lower warmer – LW - 下焦區

According to Professor Peng and Dr. Chan, Chinese Periocular Acupuncture is not just limited to the treatment of ocular diseases. The human eyes are related to every organ of our bodies making CPT very effective for stroke rehabilitation, neurological impairment, internal disorders, acute and chronic pain relief, and male and female issues. In this section, we will discuss how our eyes influence the body and how we can properly apply Chinese Periocular Acupuncture for ocular disorders, neuromuscular and musculo-skeletal dysfunction and pain, as well as the emotional and physical abuse suffered from displaying angry eye.

Diagnosis and Treatments for Five Types of Eye Dysfunctions

1. Angry Eye

- **Ocular Inspection and Diagnosis:** Angry eye (Addendum Figure 2) is also called Liver eye. It is one of the most common eye problems in our society; people from all walks of life have experienced this type of eye condition at some point in their lifetime. People suffer especially from angry eye with acute and chronic emotional trauma such as depression, frustration, irritability, overconsumption of alcohol, liver and gallbladder imbalance, joint and tendon problems, taking medications for a prolonged length of time, and emotional and physical abuses.

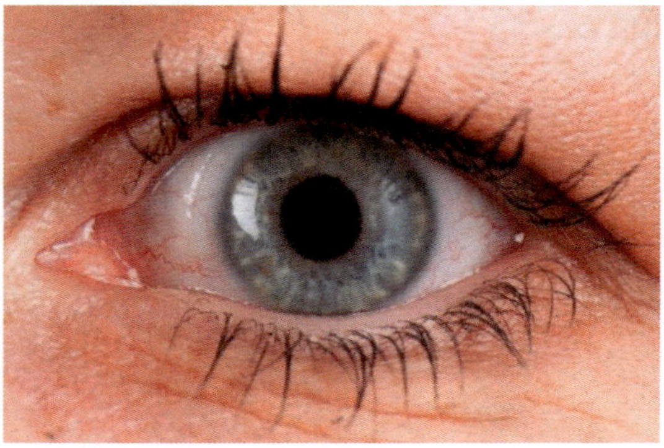

Addendum Figure 2 Angry Eye

When Liver Heat accumulates or there is Liver Heat excess, abnormal Liver Qi fires up and stirs up extreme anger which in turn will lead to red facial complexion and extreme red eye. Consequently, the eye loses its cooling element, thus causing dry itchy eye, red eye (bloodshot), vertigo, headaches with burning eye sensation. While Liver Heat not only invades the eye, it also attacks the heart with palpitations, sore mouth and lips, thirst and painful throat, kidney/bladder with dark or burning urination, stomach/spleen with indigestion, diarrhea and constipation. When Liver Blood is deficient, eye circulation is very poor and therefore it produces pale and black eye, blurred vision, floaters and flashers, and myopia. Moreover, prolonged liver stagnation can lead to chronic depression and prolonged menstrual disorders and premature onset of menopause in women.

When liver's internal tornado (Internal Liver Wind Storm) arrives, it causes rapid eye movement and painful face, neck and shoulder with red and yellow and stiff tongue. When Liver Blood is deficient, the eye's blood circulation is very poor causing eye malnourishment and eye fluid deprivation. Because of this, it produces pale and black eyes, blurred vision, floaters and flashers, and myopia. Moreover, prolonged liver stagnation can lead to chronic depression, prolonged menstrual disorders and early menopause in women.

Angry eye indicators include enlarged and red colored blood vessels covering the entire conjunctival area. Eyeballs are overstrained by intensified contraction of eye tendons and muscles. Key point: Most blood vessels are located in the Liver and Gallbladder ocuzones, and sometimes, a greenish color presents. Many patients with this eye condition often complain that the left sides of their bodies are weakening. Insomnia and fatigue are also common disorders in angry eye ailment.

- **Ocular Treatment Methods**: UW, LI/GB ocuzones, with both extra-orbital and twin needle methods alternatively. (Figure 43 and 44, page 53). Use combined inner and outer method for LV/GB region only. (Addendum Figures 3 and 4). Retain needles for 20 minutes; green tea bags may be applied for 5 minutes and eye Tuina for 5 minutes, three sessions per week.

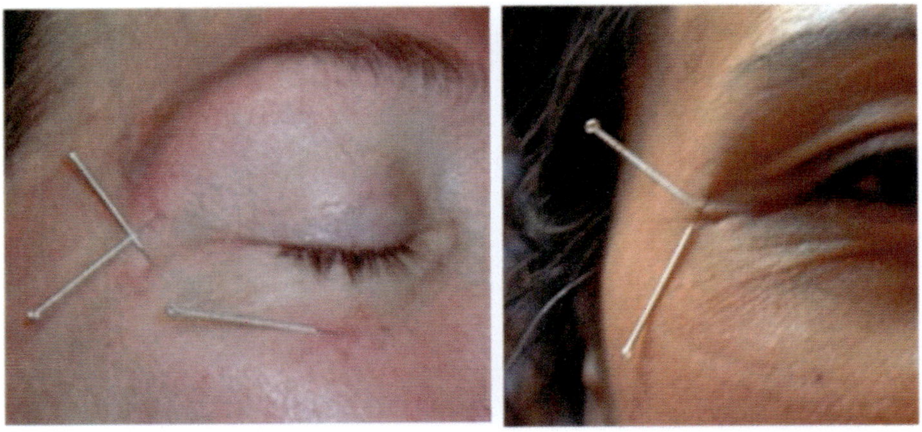

Addendum Figure 3 Extraorbital Needle Method

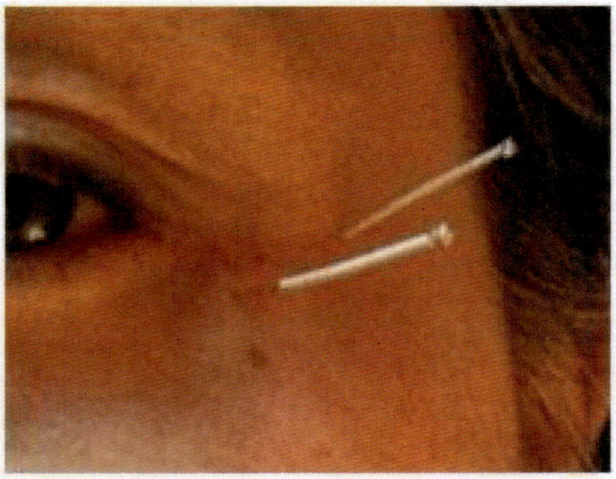

Addendum Figure 4 Twin Needle Method

- **Preventive Measures**
  1. Avoid exposure to wind especially in the spring by staying indoors when it is windy outside. The wind can affect eyes, resulting in sudden or gradual loss of vision.
  2. Consume more green colored foods and avoid spicy, sour and fried foods.
  3. Stay away from high pitched sounds, such as loud music and loud voices.
  4. Take anger management programs and seek emotional support.
  5. Avoid drinking excessive alcohol and soft drinks (high in sugar).
  6. Participate in more healthy social and family living.
  7. Develop regular hours away from computer work, reduce online gaming and time watching TV.
  8. Look at blue and green colors for a few minutes when eyes are tired; avoid looking at red and yellow colors.
  9. Resolve ongoing conflicts and identify and eliminate specific internal and external stressors.

2. Unhappy Eye

Ocular Inspection and Diagnosis: Unhappy eye is also called heart eye. Unhappy eyes are caused by an abnormal and unbalanced heart from conditions that excessively deprive the normal Yin Qi of the heart and small intestine. In other words, dysfunctions of heart eyes are manifested from experiences of prolonged excitement, strenuous workouts, sudden shock, repeated stimulation and having a constant driving force. Extreme Heart Yang excess leads to chronic sleep problems, heart attack, atrial fibrillation (AF) and loss of short term memory.

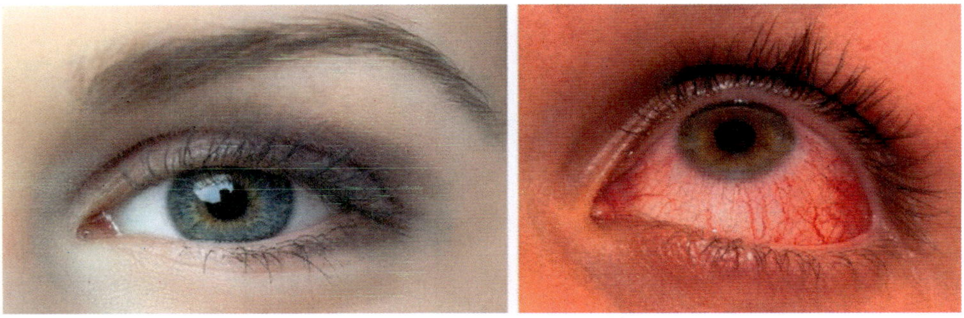

Addendum Figure 5 Happy Eye (L) and Unhappy Eye (R)

Comparing the Happy Eye to the Unhappy Eye

Extreme red eye syndrome (Addendum Figure 5) is seen by eye conjunctivitis, eye swelling, redness, excessive tearing and the appearance of abnormal blood vessels. Traditional Chinese medicine states that tears are the products of both liver and the heart. Thus, eye fluid deficiency affects the stability of liver and heart. Major symptoms such as emotional disturbances, red face, dry and sore mouth, tongue and throat, sweating, rapid pulse, vertigo, dizziness, constant thirst, constipation, difficulty in urinating and restless legs are associated with abnormal happy eyes. Moreover, an unstable heart function can also lead to uncontrollable laughing and crying which lead to pseudobulbar affect (PBA).

Abnormal Happy Eye Indicators: blood vessels generally spread over the entire conjunctival area, mostly accumulating in Heart and Small Intestine zones, sometimes with dark red color. Many patients with this eye condition often complain about three major issues: insomnia, restlessness, dry and sore mouth (red tongue at tip).

- **Ocular Treatment Methods**: MW, HT/SI ocuzones and BL1 (LW). Extraorbital method for treating HT and SI is to insert needles from HT region crossing to SI Region subcutaneously (Addendum Figure 6). Retain needles for 20 minutes; two slices of cucumber may be applied to both eyes for 5 minutes and eye Tuina for 5 minutes, three sessions per week.

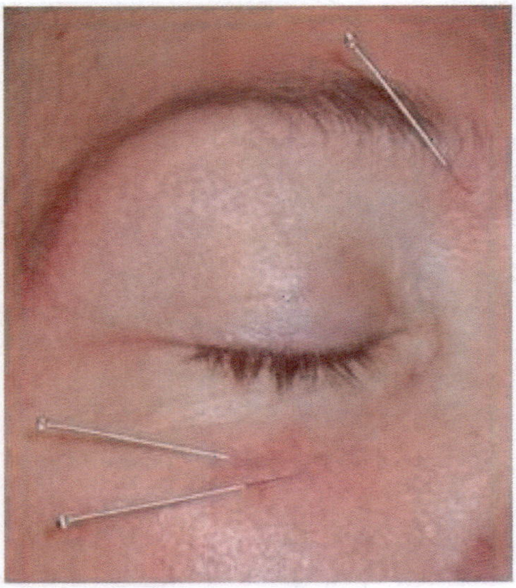

Addendum Figure 6 Extraorbital and Twin Needle Methods

- **Preventive measures**:
  1. Avoid exposing eyes to heat, especially in the summer season, staying indoors when it is very hot outside. Wearing a pair of good sunglasses is a very good way to avoid overexposure to sunlight.
  2. Consume more cool foods and avoid hot, spicy and fried foods. Gohyah tea is a tisane made from dried slices of bitter melon. It is made as a medicinal tea, and a culinary vegetable. Gohyah Tea not only is good for heart and liver, but also very helpful in promoting digestion, preventing influenza, throat inflammation and reducing blood cholesterol and body heat. It is a recommended alternative medicinal tea for patients with diabetes.
  3. Stay calm and try to reduce mental stress and strenuous physical work.
  4. Get enough sleep because good sleep is an incredible medicine for heart, eye and memory.
  5. Do not exercise at noon. A nice nap is good for both your eyes and heart.

3. Worry Eye

- **Ocular Inspection of the Eye:** It is also called Spleen eye, and is another very common eye problem in our fast-paced society. When a

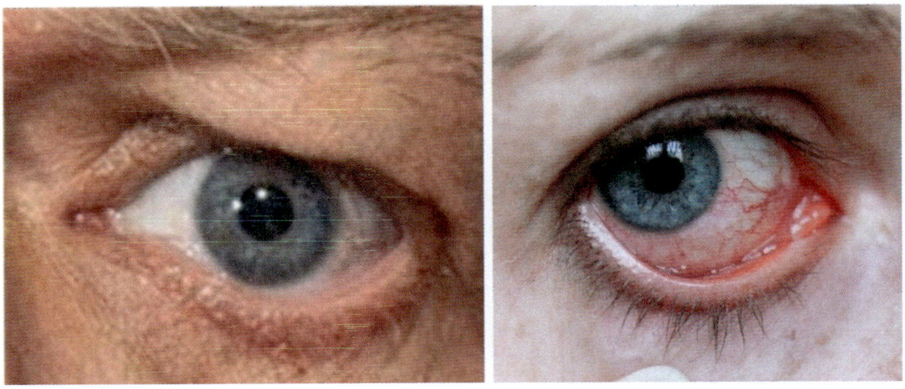

Addendum Figure 7 Worry Eye

person is anxious, worried or pensive (over thinking), imbalanced spleen and stomach can cause acute and chronic fatigue, heartburn and indigestion. Common disorders are stomach cramps, bloating, belching, and gas reflux. People with worry eye develop more winkles around their eyes, have weight gain, water retention, weakness of muscles (Addendum Figure 7). When Spleen Dampness overaccumulates, it causes secretion of water or mucus and swelling. Thus, the eye loses its cooling element. Specifically, dry eye, red eye (bloodshot), headache with burning eye sensation all team up together to cause spleen eye syndrome.

Worry Eye Indicators: Abnormally twisted blood vessels grouped near Spleen and Stomach ocuzones. Upper and lower eyelids are swollen Sometimes, yellow color may be seen around the conjunctiva near both right and left inner canthus areas. A key point to remember is that many patients with this eye condition often complain about these five major issues:

1. Upper body dampness, such as excessive phlegm discharge from lungs and stomach, heaviness of chest and upper limbs, dizziness, sore mouth and lips, coughing or vomiting.

2. Lower body dampness such as heaviness and swelling of the lower limbs. In some cases, heat and dampness team up to produce symptoms like dark burning urination, frequent flatulence, stools that smell like raw-eggs, excessive yellow vaginal discharge, and even jaundice. Wind/dampness can cause some serious joint pain and numbness of hands and feet.

3. Internal spleen dampness with serious diarrhea, tiredness, stomach cramps. A feeling of fullness or bloating, no appetite, gas and belching, water retention in the abdominal area. Colds and allergies are very common for worry eye people.

4. Some worry eye patients also exhibit myofascial skin irritation of a weepy, damp nature such as eczema, skin ulcers, and other skin allergic reactions. This is related to dampness and a buildup of toxins.

5. A "slippery" pulse and a greasy tongue coating can be felt and seen in both cases.

- **Ocular Treatment Methods**: MW and LW, SP/ST ocuzones, with both extraorbital and modified needle methods alternatively. (Addendum Figure 8). Retain needles for 20 minutes; eye Tuina for 5 minutes, three to four sessions per week.

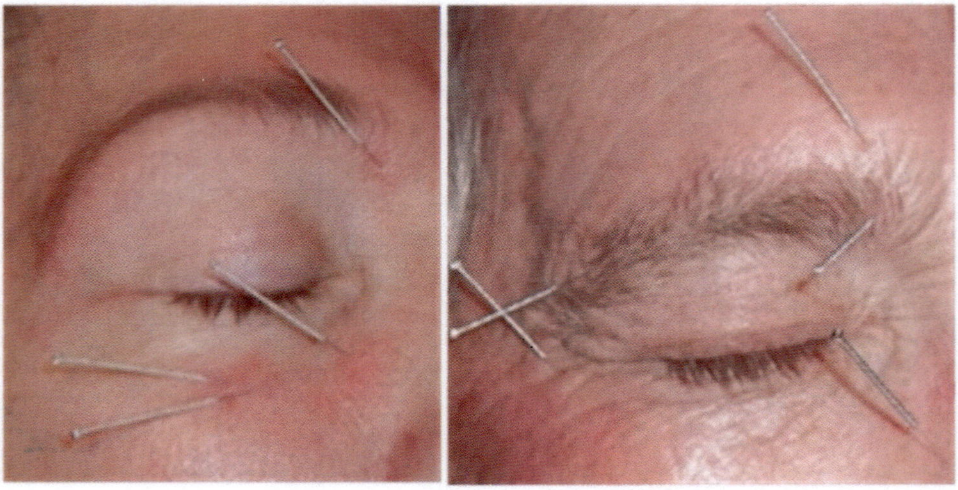

Addendum Figure 8 Extraorbital and Modified Needle Methods

- **Preventive measures**:
  1. Avoid exposure to damp weather, especially in the spring and late summer seasons, by staying indoors when it rains outside. The dampness can affect eyes resulting in sudden or gradual swelling and puffiness.
  2. Consume more yellow color foods and avoid eating cold foods, frozen products and dairy products.
  3. Stop smoking.
  4. Participate in healthier social and family gatherings, listen to soothing music.
  5. Do regular exercises and tone and relax muscles properly.

4. Grief Eye

- **Ocular Inspection and Diagnosis**: Grief eye (Addendum Figure 9) is also called Lung eye. Grief and sadness and sorrow fit in this same category. Grief eye can be seen when people experience shock and deep disbelief in situations such as death, divorce, job loss, sudden unpleasant news, feeling guilty, financial or personal loss. Grief eye affects the lung and large intestine and vise versa. One key factor is that someone with grief eye always gives up many tears and holds onto much eye muscle tension because of excessive weeping or crying.

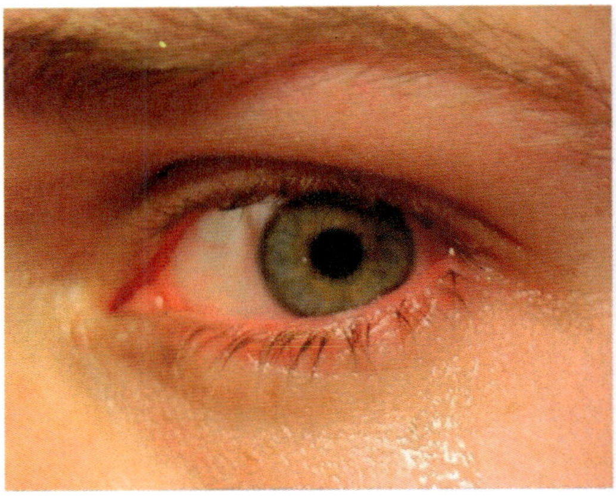

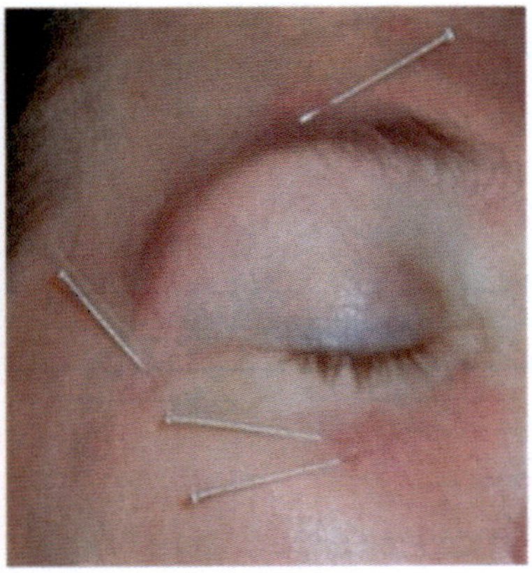

(L) Addendum Figure 9 Grief Eye
(R) Addendum Figure 10 Extraorbital and Modified Needle Methods for Treating Grief Eye

People suffering with prolonged Grief eye often experience associated lung and large intestine problems because prolonged grief depletes normal Lung Qi which leads to poor breathing and shortness of breath (asthma), coughing, urination problems, having a bad cold with running nose, allergy reactions, dry or oily skin and hair. Subsequently, an affected lung inhibits normal Qi from fully descending toward the large intestine and supporting normal fluid absorption and elimination process. Thus stagnation of large intestine Qi, fluid and Blood occurs. Many abdominal obstructions lead to intestinal dysfunction such as irritable bowel syndrome (IBS) and constipation. Prolonged grief eye can lead to the eye and body aging prematurely.

Grief Eye Indicators: Most red blood vessels are located in Lung/Large Intestine area. Dryness is one of the major complaints. Sometimes, gray color can be seen around Lung ocuzone. Insomnia, fatigue, allergic reaction, skin and hair itching, and nose bleeds are common disorders in grief eye.

- **Ocular Treatment Methods**: MW and LU/LI ocuzones + LV zone with extraorbital method. (Figure 43 on page 53 and Addendum Figure 10). Retain needles for 20 minutes; green tea bags applied for 5 minutes and eye Tuina for 5 minutes, three sessions per week.

- Preventive measures:
    1. Avoid exposure to wind, especially in fall season, and stay indoors when it is windy outside. The wind can affect eyes resulting in more dryness and tearing.
    2. Consume more white colored foods and moderately spicy foods, and avoid sour and fried foods.
    3. Seek emotional support and join group support programs.
    4. Avoid excessive alcohol and drinking soft beverages (high sugar).
    5. Morning breathing exercise is a plus for healthy lungs.
    6. Always remember this: prolonged grief is a very expensive emotion to keep and can even trigger death!

5. Fear Eye

- **Ocular Inspection and Diagnosis**: Fear eye (Addendum Figure 11) is also called Kidney eye. Fear and shock fit into the same category. Fear eye can be seen when someone gets attacked by serious illness, injuries or emotional and physical abuse. Fear eye affects the kidney and bladder and vice versa. The key factor of Kidney eye is that it also presents with a significant sign of black with gray texture around the entire conjunctival area. Qi and Blood have been deprived due to all evil pathologic factors. People who suffer with Fear eye have associated kidney and bladder problems which sometimes are brought on by dangerous situations. Special care is very much considered in Fear eye.

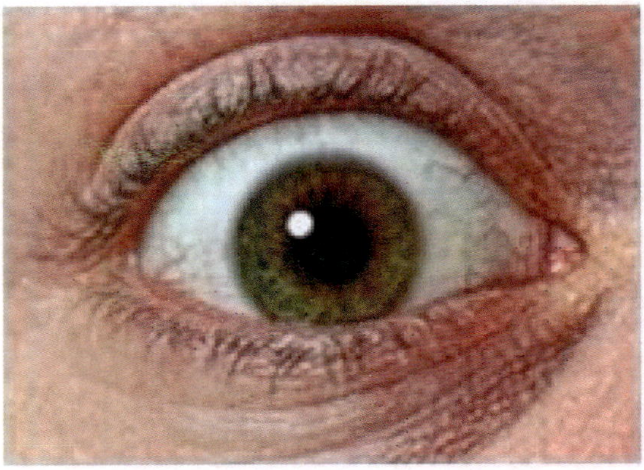

Addendum Figure 11 Fear Eye

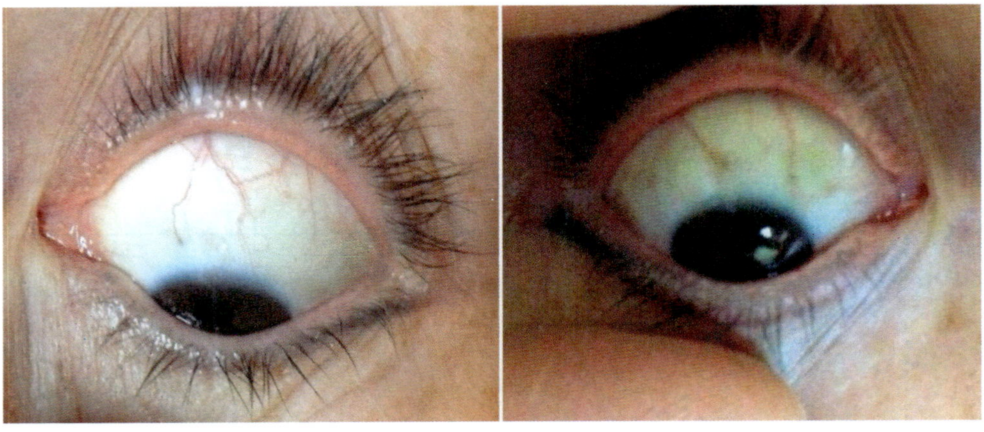

Addendum Figure 12 Capillary Changes on Fear Eye

When the kidney accumulates too many cold elements, the eye loses its important supplies of warm Qi, good circulation of blood and fluid for its muscles, vessels and skin around the eye, thus resulting in vision loss, blurred vision, floaters and flashers, myopia and other degradations of visual acuity. It also affects bladder, ears, bones, hair and vital energy. When cold invades the eye, symptoms include black and purple tongue with yellow coat, salty taste in mouth, dark or burning urination and constipation.

Fear eyes can be seen in all ages. When an adult or a child is in a fearful and shocking environment, he or she can experience overactive bladder dysfunction or uncontrolled urination or bed-wetting in children.

Fear Eye Indicators: Black eye with gray color covers Kidney/Bladder ocuzones (Addendum Figure 12). In many cases, there is a dew drop that appears at the KI/LI ocuzone. Many patients with this eye condition often complain about chills, headache, afternoon fever, nausea, diarrhea, fatigue, allergic reaction, tinnitus, joint pain, overactive bladder and lower back pain (possible kidney stones and kidney injury).

- **Ocular Treatment Methods**: MW, LW and KI/BL ocuzones (Addendum Figure 13). Also, UW with KI zones (Addendum Figure 14). Retain needles for 20 minutes; apply warm towel for 5 minutes and eye Tuina for 5 minutes, three sessions per week.

- **Preventive Measures**:
  1. Avoid overexposure to cold and dampness, especially in winter season, staying indoors when it is extremely cold and windy outside. The cold affects the eyes resulting in more painful eyes.
  2. Consume more black, blue and any dark colored foods and moderately spicy food; avoid sour, salty, and fried foods.
  3. Seek emotional support and join support groups.
  4. Avoid excessive alcohol and soft drinks that are high in sugar.
  5. Regular exercise is very helpful for persons with fear eye.

Special mention from my personal studies: Any of the above five ocular dysfunctions combined with other risk factors such as diet, lifestyle, occupational impact, sunlight effects, aging, personal and family skin history and condition, can team up to form and cause ocular melanoma.

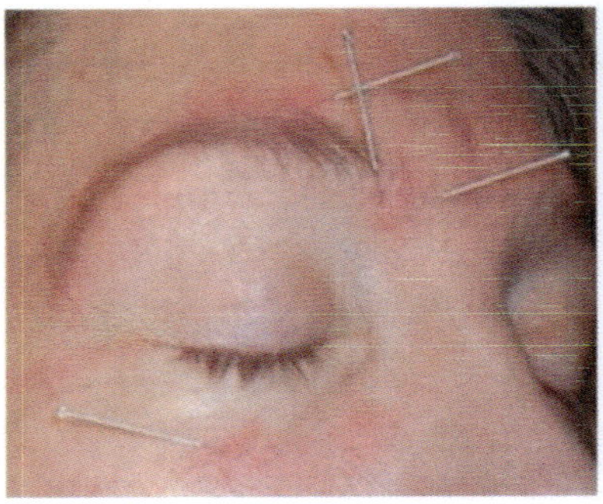
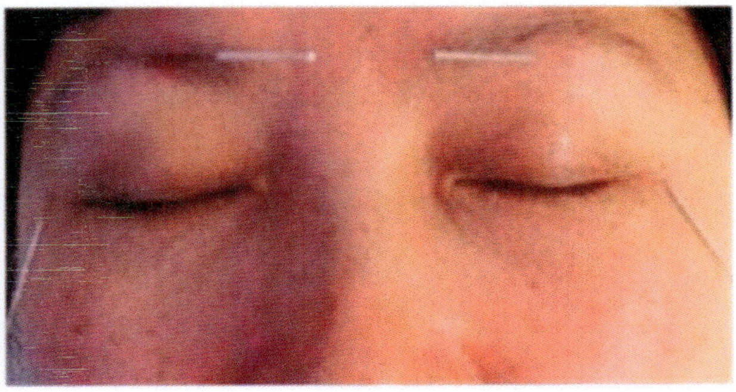

(L) Addendum Figure 13 Extraorbital and Modified Needle Methods
(R) Addendum Figure 14 Extraorbital Needle Method

Special Discussion: Periocular Acupuncture DXs and TXs for Post Traumatic Injury Syndrome (PTIS) and Stroke

- According to Dr. Chan, projecting as a dewdrop appearing in any region other than Stomach or Intestine indicates blood stagnation. For example, this may be seen in the patient who has had an automobile accident. Dr. Peng describes that projecting the dewdrop seen in Stomach and Intestine regions reveals parasitic infection. In Addendum Figure 15, the true gray dewdrops are located in this patient's right and left eyes indicating a history of kidney stones, chronic overactive bladder and chronic lower back pain caused by a history of motor vehicle accident (MVA).

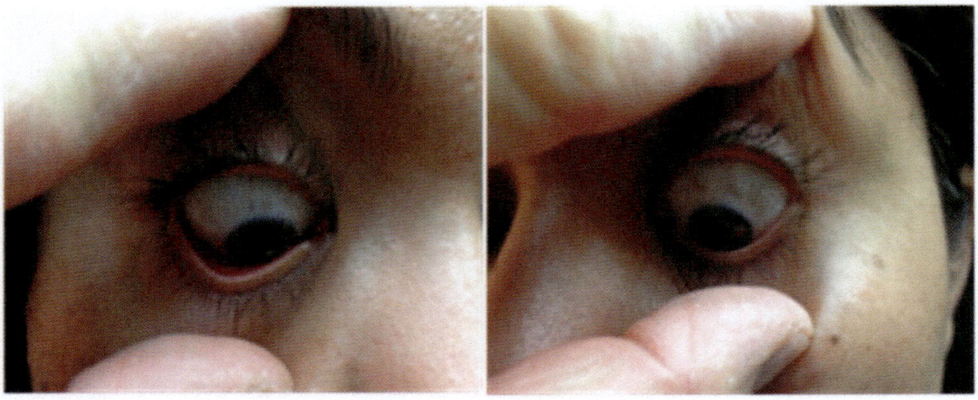

Addendum Figure 15 Projecting as a Dewdrop

- Patient with post traumatic injury with chronic lung and kidney dysfunction with fear. (Addendum Figure 16)

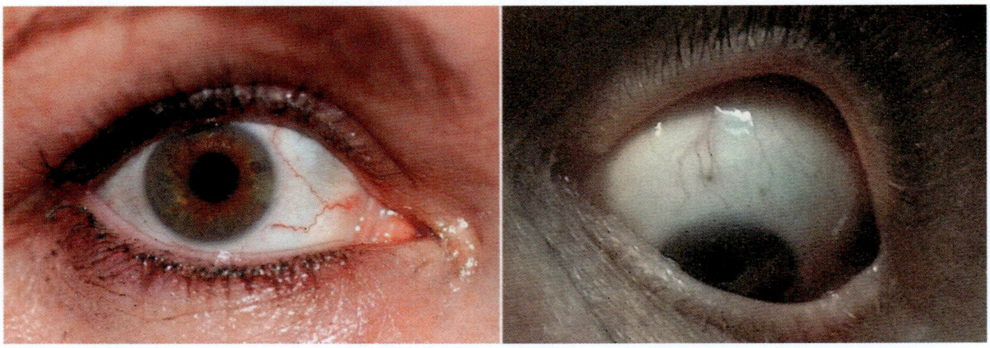

Addendum Figure 16 Capillary Changes in Fear Eye

- Patient with post traumatic injury with chronic kidney and bladder dysfunction with fear.
- Ocular treatment for patients with post traumatic injury syndromes (lower back=kidney). (Addendum Figures 13, 14, and 17)
- Patient with an acute embolic right Cerebral Vascular Accident (CVA) (Addendum Figure 18) that weakened his left upper and lower limbs. Projecting as faded gray dewdrop from Heart/Small Intestine ocuzone indicated weakness of Heart Qi and Blood stagnation (vascular dysfunction).

- In many stroke cases, treating both right and left eye's Upper and Lower Warmers along with Liver zone using inner and outer combined method and twin needle methods achieves the better result.

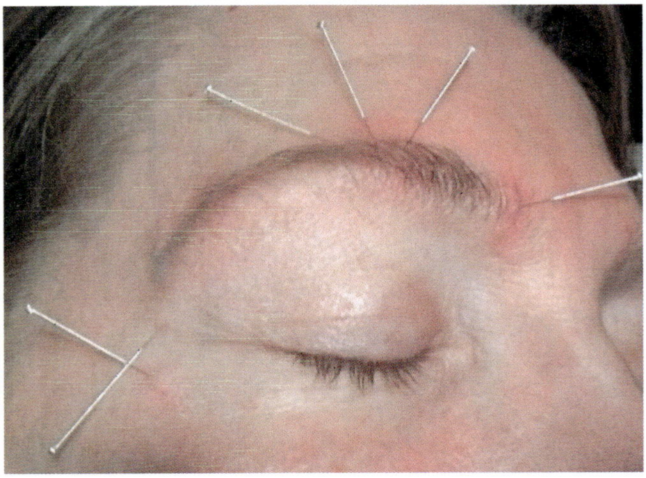

Addendum Figure 17 Fear Eye Needle Treatment

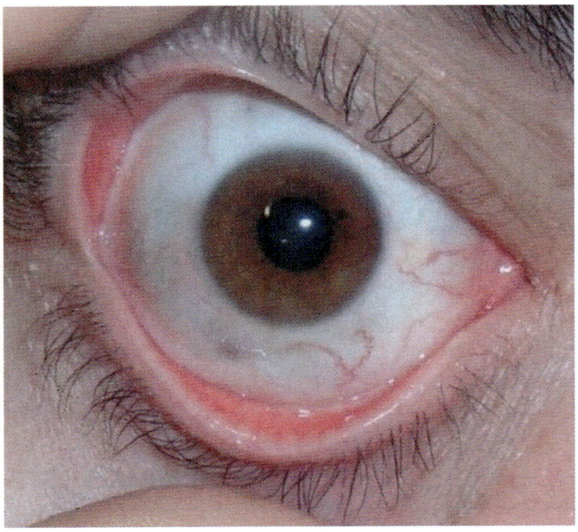

Addendum Figure 18 Capillary Changes in Cerebral Vascular Accident Patient

- Treatment Methods: Patient is placed in supine position. Select inner and outer combined method on KI/BL; extraorbital with twin needle for

UW/LI/GB, extraorbital for LW. (Addendum Figure 19). Needles are retained for 20 minutes. While CPA is in session, perform Tuina for upper and lower limbs. The treatment session ends by using the CPT Basic 10.

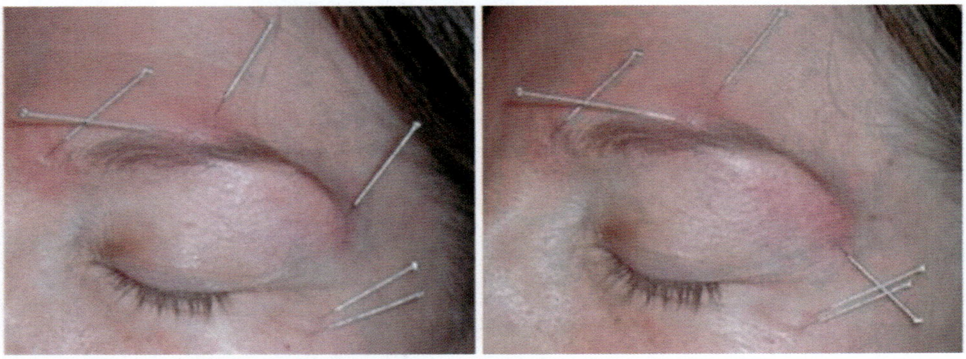

Addendum Figure 19 Stroke Patient Treatments

Always remember:

1. Strong needle manipulation is not necessary. Gently lift the needle halfway and reinsert to another angle when needed.
2. Be sure to apply pressure with a cotton ball on every needle site.
3. No CPA for patients with serious outer and inner eye injury or for patients who are extremely anxious or ill.

Chinese Periocular Acupuncture with Chinese Periocular Tuina 中醫眼周針結合眼周推拿治療法

Regular Chinese Periocular Acupuncture (CPA) with Chinese Periocular Tuina (CPT) not only helps to improve a patient's current condition, but can help patients continue to increase their own healing ability to produce dopamine in their brains. This promotes better circulation around the eyes and head in order to reduce acute and chronic inflammatory conditions and prevent more injury to their eyes, especially increasing their immune system's ability to cope with any daily stress affecting eyes and the body.

What is Chinese Periocular Tuina? 眼周推拿法

Chinese Periocular Tuina (CPT) applies various hand manipulations around the eye, face and scalp areas according to both theories of CPA and traditional acupuncture. By stimulating ocuzones and acupuncture points together, CPT can open up the meridians and unblock the stagnation of Qi and Blood, as well as balance Yin and Yang. This improves vision by alleviating eye fatigue caused by daily extensive use of computers, and prevents age-related sight loss, relaxes eye muscles, enhances blood circulation to the external and internal eyes, prevents dark eye spots, eye pouches, eye wrinkles, as well as suffering from dizziness, giddiness, soreness, nerve pain, insomnia, eye headaches or astigmatism. Using CPA and CPT together is the best approach for internal medicine and neuromuscular medicine.

Special note: Be sure to wash your hands before performing CPT.

Basic 10 Instructions

1. Press with a back and forth motion on both right and left LW/LU, LU/KI, and KI/UW with thumb and index fingers, 10 seconds and release x 3.
2. Compress SP/HT, HT/MW, MW/LV with index finger, 10 seconds and release x3.
3. Squeeze and release slowly on Yintang point 印堂 with thumb and index finger, 10 seconds and release x 3.
4. Press and knead on ST2 四白(between Heart and Middle Warmer zones) with index finger, clockwise 10 times and counterclockwise 10 times.
5. Press on Taiyang points (Ex HN 5, 太陽穴) with both thumbs and release tension with the inner surface of index finger around the orbit of eyes at the same time.
   a. Upper orbit: from Lower Warmer to Upper Warmer.
   b. Then lower orbit: from Spleen zone to Liver zone. 10 motions per upper and lower ocuzones.
6. Gently tap right and left ST8 頭維, GB4 頷厭, GB5 懸顱 and GB6 懸釐 with tips of index, middle and ring fingers for 5 times x 4 (total of 20).

7. Squeeze gently and release slowly and gently on both upper and lower orbicularis oculi, 3 seconds x 5.
8. Hold GB8 率谷 with little finger and GB20 風池 with thumb, press and release for 5 seconds x3.
9. Hold GB19 (Brain Hollow, 腦空) and GB20 (Wind Pond, 风池) with both thumbs while other fingers rest on the top of the head. Press and hold for 5 seconds x 5. Note: GB19 and 20 are excellent points for visual cortex, function of muscles/coordination of eyes. Treating these points can calm and sooth the brain/eyes and eliminate eye tension in a very short time.
10. Massage both thenar muscles of the thumbs until warm; then cup both over the eyes for 2 minutes.

The Basic 10 Illustrated

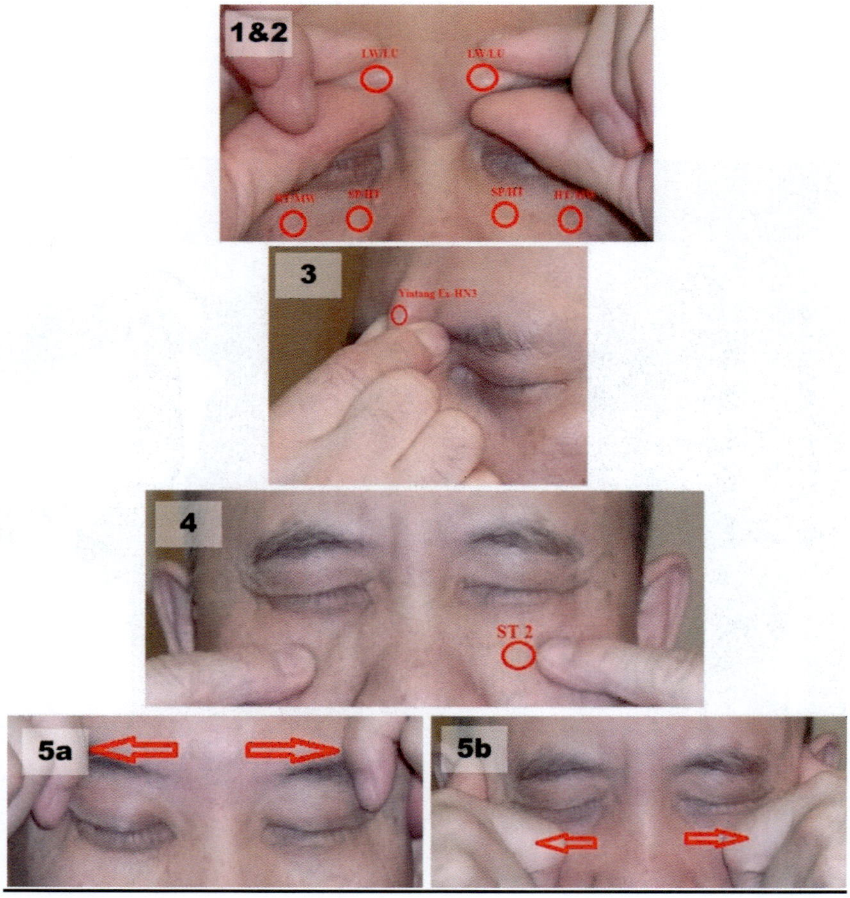

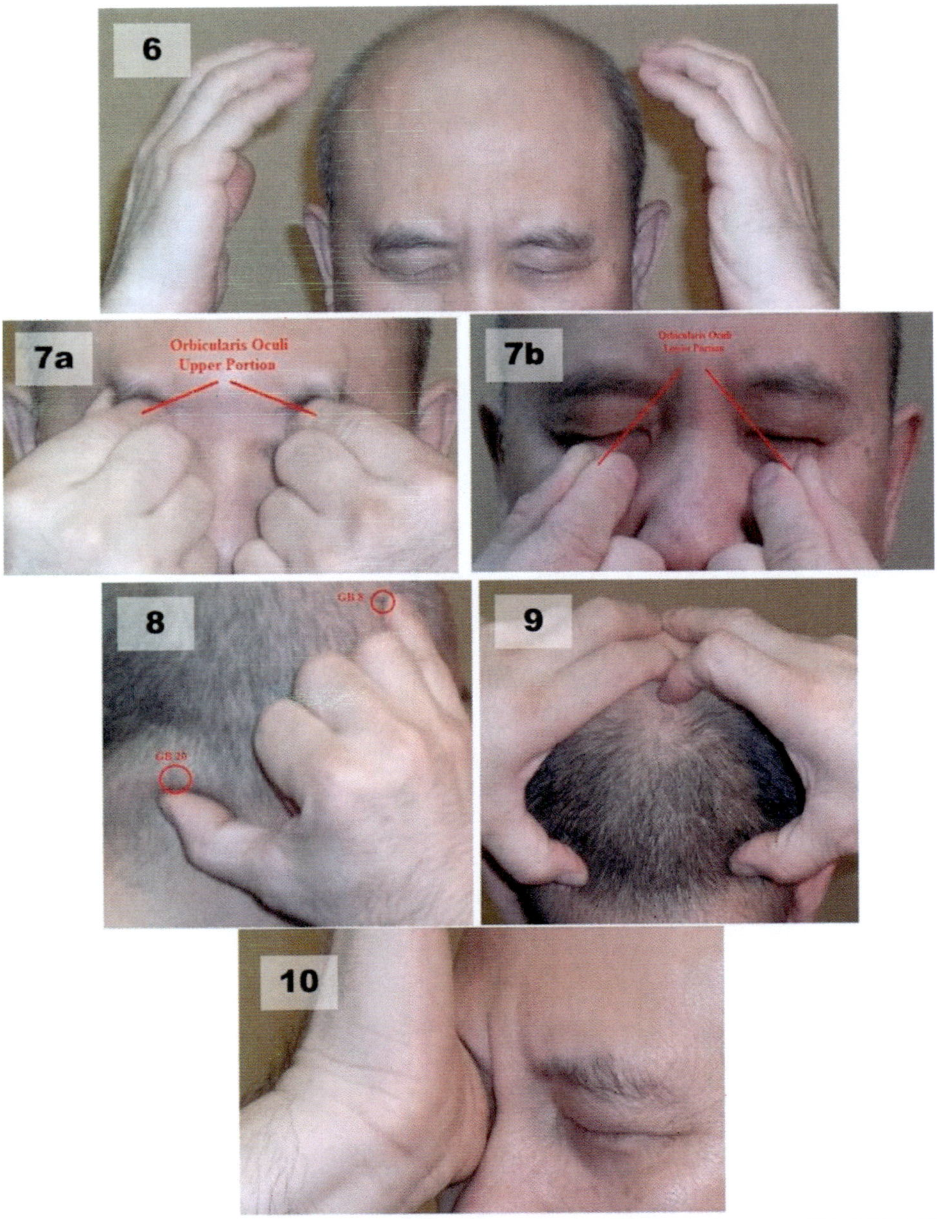

Addendum Figure 20 Basic 10 Periocular Tuina Techniques

Four Eye Passive Eye Movements, 1 Tapping, 1 Brushing and 1 Pulling to Improve Brain/Eye Health

1. Cover both your eyes with the palms of your hands and meditate for 3 minutes.
2. Open wide/close tightly and quickly for 2 seconds and repeat 5 times.
3. Close both eyes and move your eyeballs medially, superiorly, inferiorly and laterally, each direction for 2 seconds. (The eyes move together, i.e. the left eyeball moves medially while right eye ball move laterally).
4. Close both eyes and move your eyeballs clockwise 5 times slowly and counterclockwise slowly 5 times.
5. Use tapping on BL9 and GB19 for 10 times.
6. Brush the entire scalp from the front to the back, in and out with all ten fingertips for 10 times.
7. Grab and hold your hair gently to release scalp tension. Move right and left, top and back 2 times for each.

12 Important Preventive Measures for Eye Care

1. Having your eyes checked regularly with conventional or natural approaches is very crucial to your ocular health. It should be done once a year if you are over 50 or for anyone with heath concerns. Special ocular care should be taken for those who have liver dysfunction. An ocular check up is sufficient once every two years for those who are under 50 with no major health concerns. Everyone knows that ocular melanoma (OM) has affected thousands of people in the world so proper screening, testing, treatment and prevention are important approaches for those who desire to have healthy eyes.

2. Maintaining a good healthy body weight is a 'must do' lifetime duty. Watch your blood pressure, blood sugar and cholesterol levels, NO smoking or overconsumption of alcohol. Smoking and drinking can damage your eyes to a point where they cannot be repaired. Stress and depression can also lead to serious eye problems, so do something about it. It is too expensive to hold on to stress and depression because

they are 10 times worse than insomnia and can also weaken resistance to age-related eye diseases and other physical illness.

3. To have a good lifestyle, you must have a good diet. Healthy ways of eating and cooking include avoiding consuming too much sugar, salt, sodium, high fat, high calories and sour foods. Remember, because Vitamin A deficiency can impair both liver and eyes, all colored fruits and vegetables and fish are essential to your eyes. Going out to eat once in a while is okay, but cooking and eating at your home is preferred because your kitchen is the best pharmacy for your eyes. Steaming, poaching, braising, broiling, grilling, roasting/baking, slow cooking are better ways of cooking than deep frying and sautéing. Moreover, serious ocular problems can be caused by contamination from eating unhealthy processed, plastic packaged and fast foods, drinking unhealthy diet soda and other sweet beverages.

4. Avoid eye injury from bad body posture and prolonged eyestrain by keeping the proper reading distance and reading posture (always in an upright position), and reducing your TV, computer, gaming, reading and driving times. Remember the best eye and computer distance for an adult is the length of his or her arm (20"-26"). Avoid reading or watching TV in a low light condition. Always remember that according to TCM, prolonged use of your eyes can damage blood circulation. Close or blink your eye frequently to relax and refresh your eyes and reduce eyestrain. Computer Vision Syndrome (CVS) is one of the new eye diseases seen in our modern society. Proper work hours and normal sleep hours can also affect both your eyes and memory.

5. Avoid eye injury from sports and occupational and outdoor work by wearing a pair of UV protection glasses or protective goggles. Use hats to shield your eyes from sunrays. Always remember wind and sunrays are not good for your eyes.

6. To prevent eye infection, prolonged eye irritation, and eye allergies, avoid rubbing your eyes with your hands or any dirty clothes or towels. Makeup which contains a lot of chemical ingredients or bacteria that

can invisibly affect your eyelid and your eyeball, should be washed off properly. Makeup brushes, eyebrow and eyeliner pencils or brushes and eyelash tattoos, plus manmade eye falsies should also be washed regularly to protect eyes from contamination.

7. Walking 1000 steps each day or swinging your two arms up and down 100 times per day can promote blood circulation and relax your eyes.

8. Autoimmune diseases like rheumatoid arthritis can cause uveitis, type 2 diabetes or high blood pressure that can lead to age-related macular degeneration or many other potential eye problems. Having regular periocular acupuncture and periocular tuina is an alternate preventive measure for healthy eyes as well as providing wellbeing from the top of your head to your feet.

9. Report any side effects from your medications to your eye doctor if you experience a burning sensation, eye pain, itching, stinging, blurred vision, eye redness, watery eyes, oversensitivity to light, excessive lacrimation, vision loss, dizziness or excitability. Keep in mind that an overconsumption of medication can increase risk to your liver and eye health.

10. Identify triggers that often cause red and puffy eye allergic conjunctivitis such as nasal or facial skin allergies, pet dander, grass, certain trees and pollens, eye makeup, dust mites, molds. Seasonal allergies, city to city allergies, campground allergies and food allergies can also be considered.

11. Childhood obesity raises a child's blood pressure, cholesterol and occurrence of diabetes which can damage his or her eyes at an early age. So let us fight to save our younger generation by making better food choices, serving healthier foods both at homes and schools and providing more physical education programs for all ages both at home schools and public schools.

12. In my personal opinion, any improper care of our eyes can lead to serious ocular diseases as well as possible eye cancer. Therefore, it is extremely important to recharge, regenerate, replenish, renew and reimage our eyes by keeping our homes and offices clean and refreshed with some unscented candles; take time to listen to soft music and sit still in loose clothing for quiet time to distract yourself away from all stressful situations, and meditate with your heart and mind. Also, remember laughter is the best medicine for our eyes because it truly relaxes every muscle in the eyes and body, thus opening up all meridians which then promotes the smooth flow of Qi, Blood and body fluids.

Five Pathogenic Factors that Affect our Eyes Daily

1. Dryness often aggravates dry eye syndrome due to a lack of proper balance of eye fluid or tears. Prolonged conditions of dryness can cause swelling, itching, excessive tearing, burning, blurred vision, pink eye, redness, and possible sudden loss of vision.

2. Cold condition creates excessive pressure to the outer and inner eye and causes pain and black eye. Prolonged exposure to cold can gradually impair ocular health. Four common eye diseases that are closely affected by cold are retinal damage, cataract, glaucoma and age-related macular degeneration.

3. Wind causes dry eye, allergic eye (itchy, red, swollen and tearing), blurred vision, eyelid twitching and possible acute and chronic vision damage and conjunctivitis (pink eye).

4. Dampness produces excessive fluid retention within and around eyes, heaviness of eyes, bags under the eyes and swelling of the eyelids.

5. Heat and summer heat causes excessive eye fluid discharge. Red eye, dry eye and heat team up with high blood pressure and high blood sugar levels leading to progressive diabetic retinopathy (blurred vision

or darkened vision, sudden loss of vision) and conjunctivitis. Over time heat pressure can increase intraocular pressure that restricts eye mucus drainage, thus damaging the optic nerve resulting in glaucoma.

Five Impairments by Five Prolonging or Reparative Motions (五勞所傷)

1. Prolonged use of eyes impairs the blood circulation
2. Prolonged lying impairs the Qi
3. Prolonged sitting impairs muscles
4. Prolonged standing impairs bones
5. Prolonged walking impairs tendons

How Ocuzones and Acupuncture Points Relate to Eye Dysfunction

1. LU/LI ocuzone 肺/大腸區 (associated with Yuyao, 魚腰 and GB14, 陽白) the supraorbital region - blepharitis, pterygium, redness, swelling, itching, twitching.

2. KI/BL ocuzone 腎/膀胱區 (associated with Yuyao 魚腰 and GB14, 陽白) - diabetic macular edema, ocular hypertension, diabetic retinopathy, eyelid twitching, detachment of the retina.

3. Upper Warmer ocuzone 上焦 (associated with GB1 瞳子膠穴 and SJ23 絲竹空) - myopia, hyperopia, photophobia, red, dry, itching and swelling eyes, conjunctivitis, blurred vision, eye induced migraine headaches, cataracts, twitching of the eyelid, astigmatism, optic atrophy, Bell's palsy.

4. LV/GB ocuzone 肝胆區 (associated with GB1 瞳子膠穴 and Ex-HN7 球後) - eye diseases such as macular degeneration, optic neuritis, optic atrophy, pigmentary degeneration of the retina, glaucoma, early stage of cataract, myopia, astigmatism (refractive errors), ocular migraine, ocular hypertension and ocular floaters/flashes.

5. Middle Warmer 中焦 (associated with ST1, 承泣 and ST2, 四白 - retinal detachment, ocular melanoma.

6. HT/SI ocuzone 心/小腸區 (associated with ST1 承泣 and ST2, 四白) - acute and chronic keratitis, red, dry and itchy eyes, excessive lacrimation, excessive eye twitching, blurred vision, color blindness and cataracts. (Special note: ST2 is a better alternative than ST1.)

7. SP/ST ocuzone 脾胃區 (associated with B1 睛明 and Ex-HN 鼻通) - clears and expels the heat, reduces dampness, and releases the flow of eye fluid; nasal obstruction, congestion, sinusitis, rhinitis can also influence the eye's Yin/Yang and ocular glaucoma.

8. Lower Warmer ocuzone, 下焦區 (associated with B1, 睛明 and B2, 攢竹) - clears the heat and expels the wind, blurring of vision, myopia, night/color blindness, pterygium, cataract, redness, swelling and pain of the eye, excessive lacrimation, red, itchy, watery eyes. (Special Note: when needling B2, insert towards B1 for all eye diseases or Yuyao 鱼腰穴 for supraorbital neuralgia.)

More Evidence Based Findings

1. "Women with the narrowest arteries and vessels in the retina, the light-sensitive region at the back of the eye, faced nearly double the risk of heart disease" and "the study bolsters a theory that microvascular disease, the narrowing of tiny arteries and vessels, plays a more prominent role in the development of heart disease in women than in men" Associated press, by Lindsey Tanner, The AP, AZ, March 6, 2002.

2. Research at the University of Chicago Medical Center reported that disrupted sleep damages the body's ability to regulate blood – high sugar levels in the liver at night, potentially raising the risk of developing type 2 diabetes which affects eyes. Associated press, by Randoph E. Schmid.

3. Photoreceptor or ocular receptor melanopsin helps control biological clock. "Another group of researchers studied chemicals in vision nerves that are activated by light, and found that a protein they called melanopsin may act as a light-sensing pigment in the retina. Tests suggested that protein was present in retina ganglion cells, or

RGCs, which are in the nerve pathways leading to the internal clock in the brain", so these special eye cells tell the brain what time it is. 01/02/2009, A team of John Hopkins neuroscientists.

4. To prevent or control Computer Vision Syndrome (CVS)..."Every 20 minutes, look at something 20 feet away for 20 seconds" recommended by Teri Geist, OD, an optometrist in Omaha, Nebraska, and a spokesperson for the American Optometric Association.

5. Attitudes and actions can improve heath (eye health too!), "RX for wellness ingredients are optimism, accepting unhappiness, deep breathing, a dose of dirt, remembering, forgiving and forgetting, embracing novelty and the love of a pet" said Connie Midey, medical writer and reporter for Arizona Republic 08/08/2006.

6. "When it comes to powerful emotions, it is all in the eyes". Maia McCann, a professional photographer from Distracify.

7. Renata Savic, psychologist and psychotherapist explained, "Eyes can reveal even the smallest changes on the body and in the attitude of other people. Given the fact that most people are not aware of this, a skilled participant can easily get a hint on what is happening. We cannot "literally" read other people's minds in their eyes, but we can see the hints about the feelings of the person we are in contact with. These small signs change from moment to moment, and anyone can be aware of them if he or she pays attention to it".

8. "The eyes have it. Powerful photo evidence that, when it comes to expressing the gamut of human emotion, eyes say far more than words" said Skylan Harrison, 07/17/2014.

9. "My colon has something to do with my eyes?!" and my doctor said "When the freckle has a certain appearance and is found in a certain number, evidence that it is highly associated with a specific syndromes of colon polyps" Alfred Thigpen, 03/05/2012.

10. "In a new study from Tel Aviv University published in Vision Research, involuntary eye movements accurately reflect the presence of ADHD, as well as the benefit of stimulants used to treat the disorder" Dr. Rick Nauert, PhD, 08/14/2014.

11. "Ocular melanoma, OM, is an aggressive form of cancer that can involve any of three areas of the eye: the iris (the pigmented area surrounding your pupil), the ciliary body (a thin tissue layer in your eye responsible for aqueous humor production), and/or the choroid or posterior uvea (the vascular layer of the eye between the retina and the white outer layer known as the sclera; this pigmented tissue full of blood vessels nourishes the retina). These three areas are collectively known as the uvea or uveal tract, and OM can occur in any combination of the three. Iris melanomas have the best prognosis, whereas melanomas of the ciliary body have the worst. Most uveal tract melanomas originate in the choroid; the ciliary body is less commonly a site of origin, and the iris is the least common. Melanoma can also occur in the thin lining over the white part of the eye (the conjunctiva) or on the eyelid, but this is very rare." www.ocularmelanoma.org.

Again, eye health is truly an important lifesaving element for all ages. According to Wikiversity, refractive error, cataract, diabetic eye diseases, glaucoma and age-related macular degeneration are five common eye diseases in our society. If we start to educate students from our grade schools to high schools and universities, we can save and preserve eye health for our younger generation.

During the last fourteen years, I found that patients who have committed to regular preventive eye treatment have improved 70% from their chronic eye conditions. Many are able to minimize taking their medications. Their eyes and other related physical conditions are under control and pain levels are manageable. Having a more balanced life style and proper diet lead them to better quality lives they desire to achieve.

References

1. *Chinese Eye Acupuncture,* First Chinese edition by Professor Peng Jingshan
2. *Window of Health,* First edition by Dr. Hoy Ping Yee Chan OMD, L.Ac., 1996
3. *Handbook of Chinese Herbs* by Dr. Him-Che Yeung, Ph.D., OMD., L.Ac.
4. *Chinese English Bilingual Glossary of Traditional Chinese Medicine,* 1993
5. *Shiyong Zhongyi La Quan*, Chinese edition, 1991
6. Grossman, Marc, O.D., L.Ac., *Healthy Eyes with Chinese Medicine*
7. Acufinder.com/Acupuncture/Information/Detail/Healthy/Eyes/with/Chinese/Medicine
8. Rosenfarb, Andy, ND, L.Ac. "Researching Retinitis Pigmentosa (Night Blindness) with Acupuncture and Chinese Medicine" Oriental Medicine Newspaper, February, 2012
9. Chinese Medicine - www.yinyanghouse.com
10. Ocular Melanoma - Ocular Melanoma Foundation, US

If you would like to know more about Chinese ocular diagnosis and herbal medicine, please consult with *Chinese Medicine for Aging Eyes* by Hoy Ping Yee Chan, OMD and Carole Conlon, L.Ac. This book, a perfect companion to *Chinese Ocular Diagnosis and Periocular Acupuncture,* is available from Amazon.com or www.AyniWritePress.com.

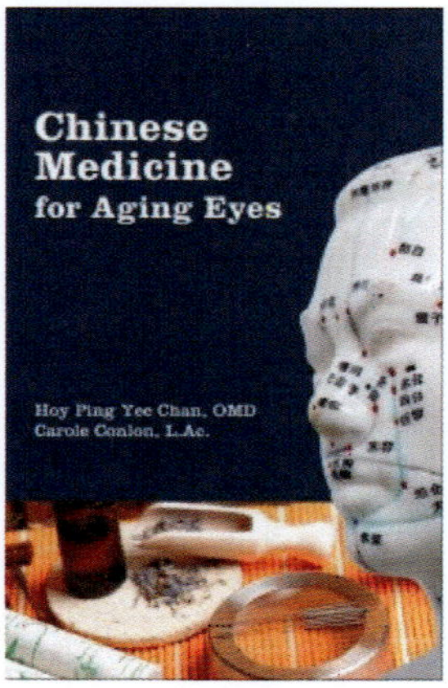

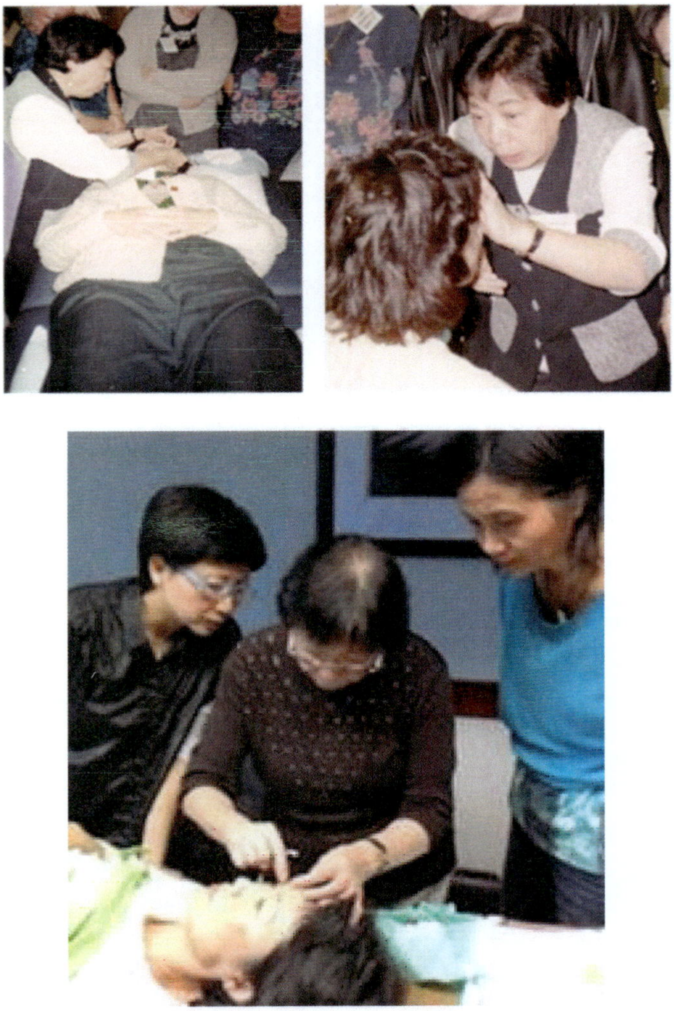

Addendum Figure 21 Dr. Chan Teaching CPA in Scottsdale, AZ, October 2000 (Top) and Demonstrating Ocular Acupuncture in Seattle, WA in October 2012 (Bottom)

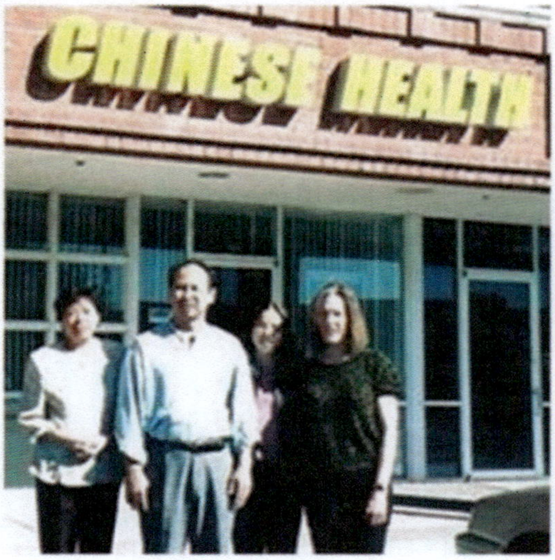

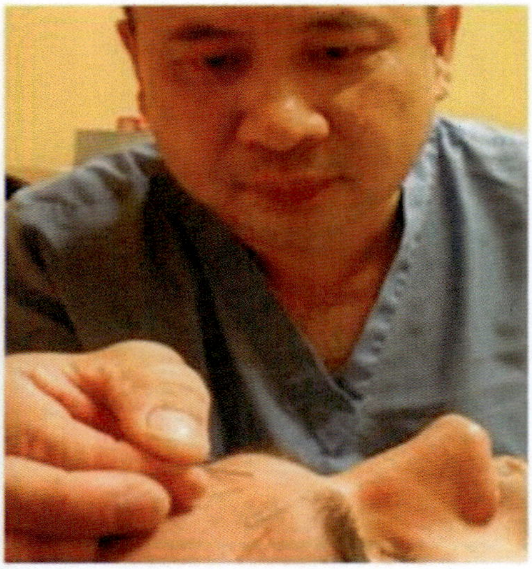

Addendum Figure 22 In front of Dr. Chen's Office, October 2000

Addendum Figure 23 Y.M.Chen, L.Ac. Providing Chinese Ocular Medicine at his Chinese Health Clinic, Anthem, AZ Since 2000

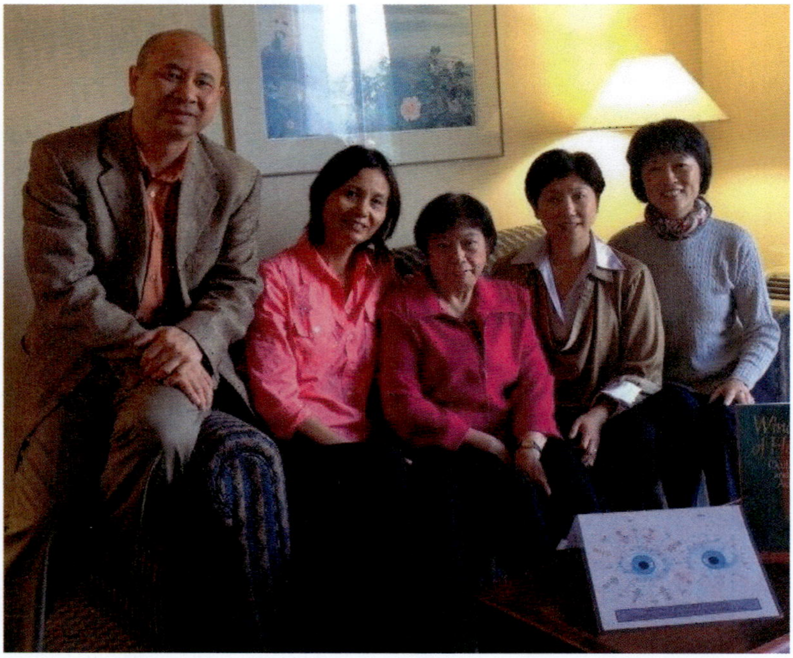

Addendum Figure 24 Dr. Chan with Chinese Periocular Acupuncturists, October 2012 in Seattle, WA , USA. From left to right: Y. M. Chen, PhD (OM), L.Ac., (Arizona), Lee Huang, MS, L.Ac. (Seattle), Hoy Ping Yee Chan, OMD, L.Ac. (Seattle), Helene Wong, PhD, L.Ac. (Seattle), Tammy Chang, MS, L.Ac. (Virginia)

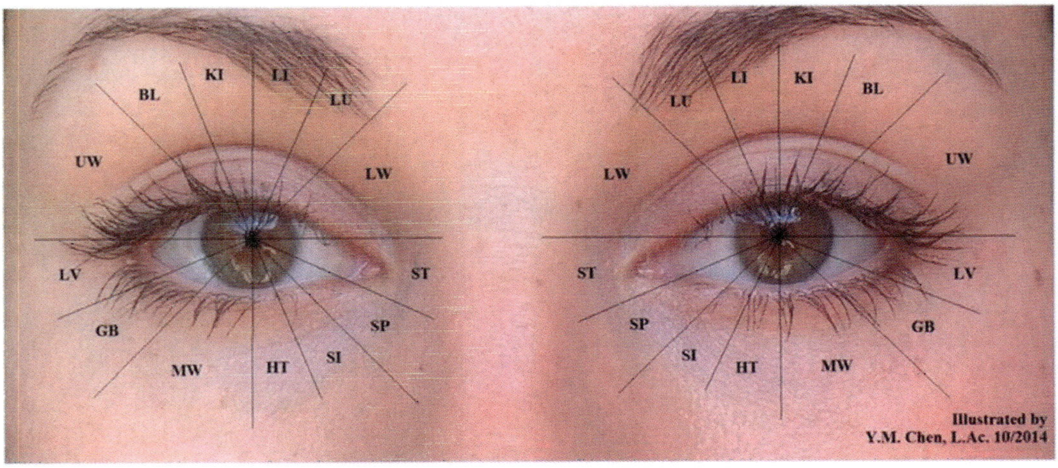

Addendum Figure 25 The Ocuzones

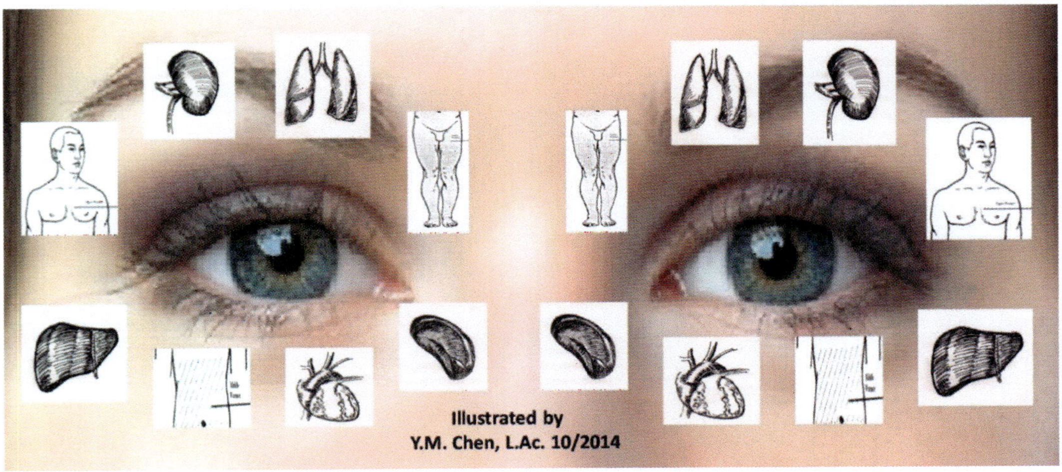

Addendum Figure 26 The Ocuzones Illustrated with Organs

Special thanks to my wife Judith Chen, my daughter Monica Chen, Lee Huang, M.S. L.Ac. MD (China), Haiping (Helen) Wong, Ph.D., L.Ac. Tammy Chang, L.Ac. for their support and encouragement. Also, my colleagues Dr. Hoy Ping Yee Chan, OMD, L.Ac. and Carole Conlon, L.Ac. for their reviewing and proofreading. Moreover, my friends and patients Alison Kalil, Haley Desmet, Mariola Sullivan and Dreamtime.com for their contribution for all eye illustrations, eye Yin/Yang symbols and CPA ocuzone chart.

Y.M.Chen, January 2015

Printed in Dunstable, United Kingdom

91220885R00071